THE 21ST CENTURY PHARMACIST

by

Billy Wease, RPh

Dear Sonya,

It is a pleasure to help you.

Thanks, Billy Wease

THE 21ˢᵀ CENTURY PHARMACIST
by Billy Wease, RPh

Transcendent Publishing
PO Box 66202
St. Pete Beach, FL 33736
(800) 232-5087
www.TranscendentPublishing.com

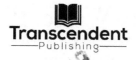

Transcendent
——Publishing——

ISBN: 978-1-7320764-7-1

Library of Congress: 2018961804

Includes bibliographic references.

Printed in the United States of America.

DEDICATION

This book is dedicated to the following:

To Jesus Christ, my Lord and Savior, who makes everything possible and pours out blessings on me daily.

To my wife, Beth, who has always been by my side and supported me in all our endeavors. You took all the supplements, cooked all the meals, did all the workouts, and everything else necessary for us to test out the components of the OptiYou RX Program. You are and always will be the only one for me and the best mother our kids could ask for.

To my children, Garrett, Olivia, and Ethan, who have put up with me demanding the best from each of you. You are all exceeding those demands and making the world around you a better place.

To you, the reader, and all people striving for optimal health, wellness, and fitness—to everyone who is becoming the CEO of your own health.

TABLE OF CONTENTS

FOREWORD

By William Cortright

I have worked in the medical field for well over three decades, and once in a blue moon you come across those unique individuals who you just know are going to shake things up. In 2014, I had the pleasure to meet one of those individuals in Billy Wease.

When you first meet Billy, you are taken aback by his country charm. He has an infectious smile and a country drawl that puts you at ease. But after just spending a few minutes with him, I could feel his passion and how he wanted to change the entire medical field for the better.

Billy told me his story of how he became a pharmacist and how he left the field to build his own brand of pharmacy. Billy created what I called a wellness pharmacy, where he would sit with patients, educate them, talk to them, and most importantly, he healed them. Billy has spent years reeducating himself to understand how to reverse disease and heal people.

I was lucky enough to work with and spend time with Billy's family. I witnessed the man in action, firsthand. I promise, *The 21st Century Pharmacist* will change your life. If you are looking to take back your health, reverse disease, get out of pain, and create permanent weight loss and health, this is the book. Billy will motivate you, educate you, and inspire you to become the best you possible.

Billy Wease is that once-in-a-lifetime teacher who will make a difference with a program that is scientifically sound and easy to follow. *The 21st Century Pharmacist* is a game changer.

—Bill Cortright
Author, Speaker, Coach

INTRODUCTION

Take Back Your Health with
The 21st Century Pharmacist

When I was 14 years old, I wanted to become a pharmacist so I could help people get well. I soon discovered that my traditional pharmacy degree did not teach me how to truly help people get well, which is why I wanted to be a pharmacist to begin with.

While I was in pharmacy school, my grandmother (Grannie) was diagnosed with cancer. Grannie was the most caring and giving person I have ever known. She always wanted to do things for me as well as all of her family, friends, coworkers, and beyond. Grannie was the best cook and made the best-tasting meals ever. Even when we tried to talk her out of cooking, she would not hear of it—she was actually offended! A dedicated hard worker, she worked her entire adult life at a sock mill. On the weekends, I would spend the night with her as often as my parents would allow. I can remember how she was always fun to be around, and her house always smelled great. She and my grandfather taught me a work ethic that is unmatched.

My love for her is immeasurable and something that is deeply ingrained in my DNA. When she was referred to an oncologist, I made the three-hour drive to take her to her appointment. Surely with my pharmacy school knowledge, I could help her make wise decisions and have an improved quality of life.

Not so much! It was suggested that she immediately begin chemotherapy and radiation. In a short time, she lost her ability to walk and control her bowels, and eventually, she was comatose until her death. Even with all my education, I could not help her have a better outcome. Something had to be wrong. I must have missed the wellness classes—except I didn't. How could I be about to graduate pharmacy school and not be able to help? This was the beginning of my awakening: that I was not going to be able to fulfill my dreams of helping people get well. I now know of many steps that could have helped Grannie realize a better outcome and fewer side effects from her treatments, but at the time, no one had ever taught me.

Grannie quickly went from the person doing everything for everyone to being bedridden and having us change her diapers. It humiliated her and totally destroyed her mentally. It was horrifying to see what the treatments did to her body. In all fairness, the oncologist told us it would be aggressive and could have side effects. We never imagined how devastating these side effects would be and how quickly they would happen.

I am convinced of two things:

1. If I knew then what I know now about nutrition and wellness, she would have had a much better life with fewer side effects, with or without her treatments.

2. If Grannie had been aware of how her quality of life would diminish from the first treatment, she would never have agreed to it. She would have lived her last days out with the cancer and seen what might happen.

Unfortunately, that seems to be the norm that my newly hired pharmacist Cole Moore experienced. He graduated from pharmacy school in 2016 and said after his internship with me that he knew less than 5% of what I teach in my OptYouRX Program. Do not get me wrong: the education in pharmacy school does prepare pharmacists to practice the standard way you are used to but with no emphasis on true health and wellness. I believe that as a member of your healthcare team, I should help you get optimally healthy. As you read more about my transformation to The 21st Century Pharmacist, you will learn that is exactly what I have helped many accomplish. Otherwise, I would not be practicing as a traditional pharmacist now.

Floyd was diagnosed with multiple tumors throughout his body. His treatment options were to see a salvage surgeon, and if the surgery was successful, he would have at least a six-month recovery. They did not expect him to live much longer than six months. Floyd and his wife decided to look for alternatives to the suggested treatment plan. I will never forget when they came into my pharmacy the first time. They had heard amazing stories of other cancer patients having success with my recommendations and were eager to consult with me. When they arrived and told me what was going on, I dropped everything and spent hours helping formulate a plan to maximize both Floyd's immune system to fight the cancer and his quality of life. I explained to this sweet couple that the plan might not offer him another day or hour, but it would provide him a better quality of life, no matter what treatment options he did or did not choose to follow. I am happy to say that Floyd did not miss any days of work for years despite being told to quit because of his illness. He had such a great attitude and felt so well, he was able to go on a mission trip to Alaska with his church. This was something he enjoyed and had been looking forward to for months but with the cancer diagnosis had been told he would not be able to go.

To you, my reader: Hi there! I'm excited that you have this book in your hands. Whether you suffer from a chronic disease, feel fatigued throughout the day, or simply want to lose weight, this is the book for you.

By optimizing your diet and lifestyle, you can create your very own personal health and wellness revolution. You'll also avoid many of the common complaints I hear so often:

- *I'm always tired*
- *I can't sleep*
- *I'm anxious*
- *I have no sex drive*
- *I have chronic pain*
- *I can't lose this stubborn fat*
- *I'm stressed*
- *I have brain fog and can't concentrate*
- *I suffer from frequent headaches*
- *I don't enjoy life anymore*
- *I take too many medications*
- *I can't lose weight*

Billy had suffered since childhood with type 1 diabetes. He was using an insulin pump and averaging over 100 units of insulin injected daily. Billy suffered with high blood sugars, neuropathy, fatigue, and muscle and joint pains, and he was overweight. He used to leave his dirty clothes on the floor and kick them into a pile so that he'd only have to bend over and put them in the hamper on wash days because it was too painful to do so daily. Mere weeks into my OptiYou RX Program, he was able to reduce his daily insulin usage to under 40 units. As he continued to follow the program and feel better, he was able to start exercising because his neuropathy and muscle and joint pains improved dramatically. Billy has now lost over 65 pounds, injects an average of 20 units of insulin daily, and can walk barefoot for the first time in his adult life. Recently, Billy's wife asked, "Why are you barefooted? I have never seen you walk through the house without shoes." Billy replied, "My feet don't hurt anymore!"

If you suffer from one or more of the above problems, this book will transform your life. I can show you the scientifically proven tools to obtain optimal health and wellness, including a lifestyle design program called OptiYou RX. The OptiYou RX Program will teach you to remake your body into a fat-burning machine, create amazing energy and vigor, and switch your brain from first gear to overdrive.

I'm Billy Wease, RPh, and this program is my brainchild. I've spent decades developing OptiYou RX. I've successfully helped countless clients overcome myriad health issues naturally, without long-term use of prescription and over-the-counter drugs. This has earned me the moniker *"The Wellness Pharmacist."*

This book shatters the health and wellness myths that keep you sick and prevent you from living life to the fullest. I'll illustrate what you need to do to stay healthy, eliminate even your most stubborn health problems, and carry vibrant health from now into your senior years.

Pat suffered with type 2 diabetes, high blood pressure, high cholesterol, achy and sore joints, general fatigue, and brain fog. He owned his own business and was concerned he would not be able to effectively continue to run and work at the necessary level if he couldn't overcome some of these issues (especially brain fog). After the OptiYou RX Program, his doctor started seeing the changes and within twelve weeks had discontinued all 21 of Pat's meds and his five insulin shots. I know this is a WOW story, but it is possible when the body is given what it needs and the toxins are taken away.

One Man's Mission to Keep You Healthy

I've used the OptiYou RX Program to help thousands of people work with their doctors and other healthcare professionals to discontinue some, if not all, of their prescribed drugs. I act as an extension of both the patient and the doctor in order to help all parties obtain the desired outcome of improved health, wellness, and fitness. As a pharmacist, I am able to work as one of three parts of the health-care triangle:

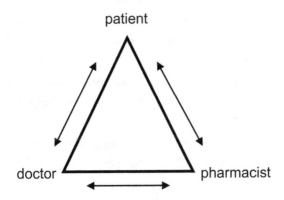

Patient, doctor, and pharmacist working as a team to create the best end results in minimal time.

I wasn't always known as "The Wellness Pharmacist." After graduating from pharmacy school at UNC-Chapel Hill, I worked for the now-defunct Eckerd Corporation drugstore chain. It didn't take me long to realize that most of the people whose prescriptions I filled were not getting well. Best case? They were simply maintained on their current medication regimen—but most of their doctors continually added more drugs to try and preserve their current (suboptimal) health status.

While working at Eckerd, I had almost no time to interact with customers or their doctors due to the emphasis that the corporation placed on volume of prescriptions filled above all else. I didn't even have time to counsel people on proper usage of their meds, much less discuss ways to improve their health. It was almost impossible to build a meaningful relationship with anyone or help solve their health problems. Helping people get well was the whole reason I had chosen pharmacy school, yet how could I help anyone without the time for a simple conversation?

After investing lots of time, money, and effort toward my education, I was weighed down with disappointment at the inability to realize my dream of helping people get well. I knew I had to take a different approach; I couldn't continue being the status quo pharmacist. It wasn't fair to my customers, and it wasn't fair to me. I knew I had to begin thinking differently to truly help people.

That's when I decided that I needed to make a change. I couldn't stand around and watch this continue to happen when I knew I could help people improve their health, given the opportunity. The first step in raising my success rate was finding an independent pharmacy where I could actually spend time talking to people and helping them resolve their issues.

I left my job with the chain and ventured out on my own, creating the first of three Prescriptions Plus pharmacies. I didn't want to be just another drug store on a corner lot—plenty of those already existed. The name "Prescriptions Plus" reflected that I was not only going to fill prescriptions, but so much more. At the time, I had no idea how much more.

Prescriptions Plus was sparked by the desire to spend time with patients, getting to know them, and discussing ways to help their specific situations. Great customer service was my highest priority, and this included giving my customers the opportunity to speak face-to-face with their actual pharmacist and create a truly beneficial relationship.

Norman and Betty were a couple that I knew I could help. This sweet, fabulous couple were my first customers at Prescriptions Plus. Both had serious health problems, and their ability to live independently was in jeopardy. Both Norman and Betty wanted to live in their home of 40 years and take care of themselves. They were both on multiple medications, and the side effects of the drugs were making matters worse. After talking with them, I studied the drug-nutrient depletions of their current prescriptions and suggested several supplements to help replenish their vitamins and minerals to a more optimal level. As a result… WOW is the only thing I can think to say here. Both had dramatic improvements in their energy, mental clarity, mobility, and overall health. They were able to live in their home for many more years, until eventually, Norman could no longer drive (Betty had never had her driver's license). After that time, as an independent pharmacist, I delivered their prescriptions and supplements after work, which allowed them to stay home a few more years.

I soon realized that this was just the beginning. I truly had no idea how huge the need for this type of service was—or how popular it would become. My customers began taking my recommendations for supplementation to minimize the drug-nutrient depletions caused by their medications, and they felt their energy and zest for life return. The word spread like wildfire.

Cathy said after only a few days of my foundational 4 supplements that she felt like a new person. Her energy and sleep were amazing, and her brain fog lifted.

More and more folks began coming into my pharmacy for advice on supplements and information on how to minimize the possible side effects of their medications. I knew I had to continue learning how to help people be healthy and feel great through natural health and supplementation.

Modern Western medicine offers few choices for patients: pharmaceutical drugs or operations and procedures. Those seem to be the final answer. But with no discussion of our lifestyles or the factors that contributed to the problem in the first place, how can we ever become well? Prescriptions Plus pharmacies operate under the belief that medications are a temporary tool, like stitches or bandages—useful for a finite period of time, until we correct the problem by changing our habits through lifestyle reconstruction. Ideally, the right treatment soon fixes the underlying problem and renders medications and drugs unnecessary.

Think about it: if your car tire picks up a nail and develops a slow leak, you have two options:

1. Add air multiple times daily.
2. Remove the nail and have the tire repaired.

The slow leak in a tire is like your health problems. Taking a prescription drug without addressing the cause of the problem is like adding air to that tire instead of simply fixing the leak. If you ignore the damage to the tire, it gets worse over time, and more air will be necessary each time to get you where you're going. Likewise, not resolving the cause of your health problem leads it to become worse, possibly triggering more conditions that will bring with them multiple prescription drugs and their side effects—all of which ultimately does nothing to fix the core issue.

Prescription drugs are like putting a Band-Aid on a bullet wound. Sure, it masks some of the symptoms, and things look better on the outside, but beneath the surface, that wound continues to fester and slowly deteriorate until things are out of control. That is not the future of health care.

Chad came to me and said he needed help. He had Crohn's disease and was unable to eat any of the foods he enjoyed without severe stomach pain and diarrhea. Even the multiple medications he was on provided no relief. I talked to Chad about how inflammation in the gut could be causing many if not all his problems. I made Chad a supplement regimen that included the foundational 4 (he especially needed digestive enzymes) and gave him a list of foods to eat and foods to avoid. Within just a few days, Chad said it was a miracle, and he was working with his doctor to reduce his medications. A month later, he was off all medications and was eating the foods he enjoyed again with no problems. Today Chad remains pain- and medication-free and feels and looks great. This is due to fixing the cause of the problem rather than covering up the symptoms with prescription drugs.

Knowledge Is Power

I continued my education and obtained an advanced fellowship in Metabolic and Nutritional Medicine from the Medical Metabolic Institute through the American Academy of Anti-Aging Medicine (A4M). My family and I felt great and enjoyed robust health as we adopted the lifestyle changes I was learning. My wife and I wanted everyone to experience the same benefits, regardless of age or current health condition. That led me to begin creating the OptiYou RX Program.

By reading this book, you are beginning a journey. You'll discover how the lifestyle changes taught in OptiYou RX can help you create long-term optimal health, wellness, and fitness. You have the power to take your health back, and you'll realize this as you read more testimonials from some of the people who have used OptiYou RX to overcome serious health problems without the use of prescription drugs. Many of these people were told that they would be maintained on drugs forever, that there was no cure for their condition, or that they were just getting old and ailments were to be expected. **That wasn't true for them, and it doesn't have to be true for you.**

I will show you exactly how to feel better than you've ever felt before. For example, meet David. David was a diabetic most of his adult life and suffered with overweight issues, high blood pressure, high cholesterol, and of course, high blood sugars. These health conditions persisted despite the treatments and diabetic training David was following. At age 60, he had a heart attack that required bypass surgery. This was a wake-up call, and David and his wife decided it was time for a change to a healthy lifestyle. David was tired of sticking insulin via needles into his body four times daily to control his blood sugar. He was told there was nothing he could do to reduce or eliminate his insulin shots. The medical experts said he was too old, and this state of affairs was just something he needed to accept. After beginning my OptiYou RX Program, he was able to work with his doctors to discontinue not only all of his insulin shots but also his metformin, blood pressure, and cholesterol medications. David and his wife now do CrossFit multiple times a week, and he feels and looks great.

CHAPTER 1

Healthcare in America:
What All Consumers Must Know
to Survive and Thrive

What if everything you've learned about healthy eating and weight loss was *wrong?* What if science actually says something different than what you've been taught? What if fat isn't the fiend it's been made out to be?

Sylvia came into my pharmacy with a laundry list of conditions— and little hope. At age 37, she had been on medications and insulins for years. She took four insulin shots daily and was scheduled to begin dialysis shortly after our consult. Within just one week, she had cut three of her four insulins down to 1/3 of her previous dosage and eliminated the fourth shot altogether. Her fasting insulin number went down over 100 points in just days. Shortly, she was able to completely discontinue three of her four insulin shots and only used 1/3 of the dose for the other daily insulin shot. After nearly two decades following various snippets of mainstream medical advice, Sylvia accomplished all this by embracing the high-fat diet and using the four foundational supplements of my OptiYou RX program.

Not many Americans implicitly trust the news media regarding politics. I encourage you to entertain a similarly healthy level of skepticism about diet, nutrition, and health. Question what you read in newspapers, magazine articles, or social media posts. Take the soundbites you hear on radio or television with a hefty grain of salt. If you wish to be truly health-conscious, it is important to properly process the information you're fed.

Question funding, motivation, and quality of research. When it comes to something as important as your health, only take your information from the true experts, not someone on a video who may have no real training or education. Your health is your most important asset.

The dietary misinformation that has been perpetuated for decades is costing the world dearly in lives lost. Just look at these sobering statistics from the American Diabetes Association (ADA):[1]

- In 2012, 29.1 million Americans (9.3% of the population) were diagnosed with diabetes. The majority of these cases are type 2 diabetes, a disease characterized by both high blood sugar and obesity, which can be prevented (and in some cases reversed) by lifestyle changes. More on this later.

- 25.9% of all seniors (11.8 million) suffer from either diagnosed or undiagnosed diabetes.

- 1.4 million Americans are diagnosed with diabetes each year.

- Diabetes is the 7th leading cause of death in the U.S.

A study published in the medical journal *JAMA* found that a startling **50%** of all Americans have either diabetes or prediabetes.[2]

Other facts about diabetes are equally disturbing. In 2012, the ADA said that 86 million people age 20 and up had prediabetes—up from 79 million just two years prior in 2010.[1] Of those with prediabetes, it was estimated that up to 30% will develop type 2 diabetes within five years.[3] The risk of death for adults with diabetes is 50% higher than for those without diabetes.[3] This is because those with the disease are at higher risk of serious health issues including blindness, kidney failure, heart disease, stroke, and the loss of toes, feet, or legs. Diabetes is the leading cause of blindness, kidney failure, and amputations below the waist in the U.S. The cost of diabetes is astronomical at $245 billion per year.[3]

The news doesn't get much better for kids. According to the ADA, approximately 208,000 youths under age 20 have diabetes.[1] The incidence of type 2 diabetes mellitus as well as two prediabetic conditions (impaired fasting glucose and impaired glucose tolerance) among youths has been rising.[4,5]

A decade ago, less than 3% of all newly diagnosed cases of adolescent diabetes were type 2. The remaining were type 1, a condition that is much harder to predict or prevent. Today, 45% of adolescent diabetes are classified as type 2 diabetes, coinciding with the epidemic of childhood obesity.[5]

Obesity encourages a condition known as **insulin resistance,** wherein the body ignores blood sugar-lowering signals sent by insulin to the brain. Insulin resistance precedes the development of prediabetes and type 2 diabetes—meaning those who are insulin resistant are more likely to develop these conditions. Insulin resistance by itself does not actually *cause* type 2 diabetes, but it plays a starring role in the development of the disease by causing the cells that produce insulin (pancreatic beta cells) to work overtime. In prediabetes, these beta cells are no longer able to make enough insulin to prevent insulin resistance. This causes the blood glucose levels to skyrocket above the normal range.

In obese children, insulin resistance progresses to type 2 diabetes much faster than in adults.[5] Sadly, developing diabetes early in life highly increases the chance of these children suffering from cardiovascular problems at an early age.

Diabetes isn't the only consequence of being overweight or obese. Putting on extra pounds also increases risk of **nonalcoholic fatty liver disease (NAFLD),** which an estimated 80-100 million Americans suffer with.[6]

NAFLD happens when too much fat builds up in the liver. As time goes on, those who have NAFLD can develop a serious form of the disease known as nonalcoholic steatohepatitis. This condition causes damage similar to that inflicted by years of heavy alcohol abuse. This damage includes liver inflammation, which may lead to scarring and damage that can't be reversed. In many cases, the eventual result is cirrhosis and liver failure.

Luckily, our bodies have the ability to reverse insulin resistance and some of its associated problems. Remember David? He came to see me as a last resort. He was very upset with his condition and treatments. He was taking prescription medications to treat diabetes, high cholesterol, and high blood pressure. He had a large blood clot in his leg and ankle that had been there for years and appeared black. The swelling made it impossible for him to put on his own socks. Despite constant medication and exhaustive standard treatments, David's numbers never got any better, and he was fed up.

I told David about the OptiYou RX Program, which was starting a session the very next day. David signed up immediately. On my recommendation, he had some blood drawn to test his fasting insulin—a test his doctor had never ordered. The results were clear: David had extreme insulin resistance and inflammation, which were certainly contributing to his poor health.

Within three weeks, David called me. He was cackling with laughter. While washing dishes after dinner, he'd turned from talking to his wife back to the sink, and **WHOOSH!**—his pants fell clean off. He'd lost so many inches, he had to buy all new clothes. By the end of 12 weeks, David's blood pressure, blood sugar, and cholesterol had all normalized, and his doctor had discontinued all his medications. The blood clot on his leg returned to his normal skin color, and he lost all swelling. David was ecstatic to be able to put on his normal socks again.

Too Much Emphasis on Treatment Rather than Prevention

The obesity epidemic can be at least partly blamed on the health and diet misinformation perpetuated from every corner in America today. It may be difficult to believe, but 16.9% of American children and 34.9% of adults—**one-third** of all grown people!—are obese.[7] Although it is said that we have one of the best health-care systems in the world, Americans are fatter and sicker than almost every other First World country.

The conventional healthcare system has adopted an approach of disease management rather than disease prevention. It ignores the critical role that diet plays in health and is focused almost exclusively on treating—rather than **preventing**—disease. Mammograms and colonoscopies are ordered to detect existing cancers, but little priority is given to lifestyle changes that could prevent cancer development in the first place. Drugs are used as the first line of defense against America's number 1 killer, heart disease, and its contributing factors such as high cholesterol. If patients are given any advice at all, it's to lower the fat in their diet without regard to the *kinds* of fats they consume or the amount of sugar they take in.

The Cholesterol Myth

As a consequence of the rise in obesity and diabetes, heart disease prevalence is also steadily rising in the U.S.[8] By 2030, 40.5% of the U.S. population is projected to have some form of cardiovascular disease. This is up from 37.8% in 2015.[7]

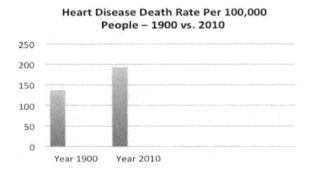

In 1900, people ate a very different diet than what we consume today. Since then, heart disease death rates have risen from 137.4 per 100,000 people to 192.9 per 100,000 in 2010.[9]

Heart disease is the #1 killer in our country today. Consider these alarming facts from the Centers for Disease Control (CDC):[10]

- 610,000 people die of heart disease annually in the U.S.—1 in every 4 deaths.
- The most common type of heart disease, coronary heart disease, is responsible for 370,000 deaths each year.
- Approximately 735,000 Americans have a heart attack each year.

The general public holds certain ideas as absolute "truths"—things like the direct link between high cholesterol and heart disease or that we can avoid heart disease by eating a low-fat diet with minimal saturated fat. **This is hogwash!** The thought of cholesterol contributing to heart disease is one of the biggest myths that the American public has been falsely led to believe over the years.

In *The Great Cholesterol Myth,*[11] Dr. Steven Sinatra, America's leading integrative cardiologist, has this to say about the supposed link between high cholesterol and heart disease:

- High cholesterol by itself has not been proven to cause heart disease.
- Cholesterol alone is a poor predictor of heart disease.
- Only around half of heart attack victims have high cholesterol.
- Statin drugs (used to treat high cholesterol) may play a role in diabetes.[12] Despite studies that claim statins may decrease the risk of Alzheimer's disease, there are reports of patients developing dementia after taking statins. *[Note: switching from a fat-soluble (lipophilic) statin to a water-soluble (hydrophilic) statin may reduce the risk of memory problems associated with statins, which is why it's a good idea to work with both your doctor and a knowledgeable pharmacist to determine what medications are best for you.[13]]*
- Chronic inflammation is a significant predictor of coronary artery disease. High levels of C-reactive protein (CRP) can indicate high amounts of inflammation in the body. High levels of CRP are associated with a doubled risk of death from heart disease when compared to the risk linked to high cholesterol.

That last point is one you likely won't hear about at your next heart checkup.

When a patient named Janie began my OptiYou RX program, her CRP was over 39—I teach that 1 or less is optimal. She had fatigue, weight gain, and other health issues, which is why she chose to come to my free OptiYou RX Wellness Workshop to learn more. Janie's doctor referred her to the program, and here is her dramatic transformation in her own words:

> My name is Janie, and I am 63 years old. It was in August that I made the decision to make a radical change in my health and lifestyle. I was 40 pounds overweight and experiencing lots of fatigue. I had been blessed to avoid prescription medications and desired to stay on that path. With that hope and desire, I began seeing an integrative doctor in July. She recommended I attend the OptiYou RX Wellness Workshop and Summit that would be held in her office the very next month.
>
> Billy suggested an extensive blood panel that he created to measure some of the most important markers for optimal long-term health. All of my results seemed to be in a normal range except my C-Reactive Protein (CRP) and vitamin D levels. The CRP tested at a very high 39.56 and indicated I was at an increased risk for a future cardiovascular event. My vitamin D was a lowly 20.4.
>
> The OptiYou RX Program fit into my lifestyle and increased my energy. My results in 12 weeks following the program were unbelievable. I lost 17.2 pounds of fat and had a radical change in my bloodwork for the better. Eating great-tasting, healthy food, taking quality supplements, drinking alkaline water, and participating in a fat-to-muscle exercise program was not only easy, but it brought my CRP down from 39.56 to 1.0 in only 12 weeks.
>
> My results were so amazing that my husband signed up for the OptiYou RX Wellness Summit in January, and I decided to take the program again with him. Billy teaches so much information that I knew I could learn more and support my husband Rick. Rick had been on cholesterol medications for

over 10 years, and he wanted to learn how to get off his medicines. His high density lipoprotein (HDL) level was low and declining while low density lipoprotein (LDL) was high. This is exactly the opposite of what the doctor and Rick wanted. After learning of Rick beginning the program, his doctor took him off the cholesterol medication and retested his cholesterol levels 12 weeks later. His HDL increased for the first time since being tested, and his doctor was happy with his numbers and told him he could stay off the medications.

I want to thank Billy Wease for his OptiYou RX Wellness Program and his dedication and hard work in developing a program that allows him to use his God-given talents in saving lives and improving health. He truly has a servant's heart and cares for all his clients who join his program. God has blessed him, and may God continue to bless him and all those who have turned their health around with all the science and knowledge, supplements, and all the other necessary tools he gives participants in his program. It produces real life-changing results in people's health and has saved many lives.

We're constantly told to avoid fat and eat a low-fat diet, without being warned away from the true culprits of heart disease: **sugar** and **high-fructose corn syrup.** Eating these causes inflammation in the body, making you vulnerable to heart disease and just about every other disease known to man.

The low-fat food craze can be traced by to the 1950s, when President Eisenhower suffered a heart attack. Around the same time, a Russian researcher named David Kritchevsky released a study on the impact of cholesterol consumption in rabbits. In the study, rabbits fed a vegetarian diet with added cholesterol developed artery-clogging plaques.[14] Kritchevsky performed more experiments on rabbits and reached the same conclusions.[15,16]

The results were distributed and accepted without consideration to the fact that rabbits normally eat a vegetarian diet. Adding fat and cholesterol to a rabbit's diet has considerably different consequences than for humans, who are natural omnivores.

In the mid-1970s, high-fructose corn syrup (HFCS) was introduced to the U.S. It wasn't long before this product, originally discovered in Japan, appeared in everything from ketchup to cereal to mayonnaise to baked goods—pretty much anything that called for sugar. People were told that low-fat was healthy—even if those low-fat foods contained HFCS or sugar.

Sugar is *anything but* healthy. Recent research has found consistent evidence among studies that sugar intake is linked to cardiovascular disease.[17] In fact, the researchers found that sugar intake was a more significant risk factor for heart disease than fat or salt consumption.

High-fructose corn syrup is no friend to the body, either. HFCS contributes to heart disease and NAFLD more quickly because it actually causes *more* fat to build up on the liver than sucrose (table sugar).[18]

Adolescents who drink beverages sweetened with HFCS are more likely to develop insulin resistance and are fatter around the waist than those who do not.[18,19]

Perhaps most disturbing about added sugars is their propensity to reduce the body's ability to use nutrients from foods eaten at the same time. Added sugars also steal nutrients from body stores.[20,21] This is because the oxidation of sugar requires certain nutrients such as riboflavin, other B vitamins, and niacin.[20,21] Worse yet, eating added sugars damages mitochondria, the powerhouse of your cells, interfering further with energy production.[20,21]

There is simply **nothing** good about sugar. Avoid it at all costs!

Many of the studies that purport HFCS has no impact on heart disease risk or obesity were conducted by researchers who had a conflict of interest. One author responsible for multiple studies receives consulting fees from the fructose/sucrose/HFCS industry, incentivizing him to prevent personal financial loss by avoiding incriminating the deadly sweeteners.[22]

They Said It Was Safe

Always question what you're told. Is it the truth, or is the statement designed to line someone else's pockets? For centuries, people were told mercury dental fillings were safe (some weren't even told that dental amalgams contained mercury at all), and now many are walking around with a toxic chemical in their mouth. The worldwide jury is still out on whether dental amalgams are dangerous, but many professionals have questioned their safety.

A study published in December 2016 indicates that there is cause for concern. Researchers found that amalgam fillings were linked to higher levels of mercury in the blood of 14,703 subjects.[23]

Would you advise a pregnant loved one that an amalgam filling was a good option for her? If you don't see a problem with that, would you recommend the swordfish for her at your dinner out? The Food and Drug Administration (FDA) suggests that pregnant women and women trying to conceive limit exposure to fish and shellfish that contain higher levels of mercury such as swordfish and king mackerel.[24] Despite this caution, the FDA has not followed in the steps of other countries like Denmark, Sweden, and Norway by banning mercury amalgam fillings. In fact, the FDA is adamant that they are safe.

Mercury from dental fillings also contaminates wastewater, meaning that mercury ends up in your drinking water and food supply.

You must also avoid mercury in your supplementation. Do not underestimate the importance of consuming adequate amounts of the fish-sourced essential fatty acids EPA and DHA for fetal health and childhood neurological development. Quality fish oil supplements have been tested for toxins such as mercury and polychlorinated biphenyls. There is no such thing as organic ocean water, and as the platitude states: "You are what you eat from your head to your feet." This applies to the foods we eat as well. Fish are exposed to toxins from all sides, so when we consume untested, low-quality fish products, we are poisoned by what they ate.

Have you ever questioned whether fluoride is actually good for you? You should. Fluoride competes with iodine for uptake by the thyroid gland and other tissues in need of the mineral. The damage is considered so bad that most of Western Europe does not fluoridate their water supplies.

A study published in April 2016 found a direct correlation between fluoride exposure and lower IQ scores in children.[25] Another study from 2015 concluded that children drinking water with high levels of fluoride had significantly lower overall IQs than children drinking water with low levels of fluoride.[26] And yet, flavored fluoride treatments are a mainstay at dental visits!

Fluoride exposure also increases the formation of the bone-destroying cells called osteoclasts and speeds up bone loss in postmenopausal women.[27]

Iodine: Why Table Salt Isn't Enough

Another myth you may believe is that you take in adequate iodine in your diet. Iodine was first added to table salt in the 1920s in order to prevent goiter (enlargement of the thyroid gland).[28]

Despite this addition, iodine deficiency is still all too common. According to World Health Organization (WHO) guidelines, a population's mean urinary iodine levels should exceed 10 µg/dL, and no more than 20% of the population should fall below 5 µg/dL. Between 1971 and 1994, median urine iodine levels in the U.S. fell by 50%.[29] A 2002 study showed that iodine levels had not improved since 1994.[30]

Iodine deficiency occurs for a number of reasons. The government-mandated addition of iodine to table salt does little good when the same government now warns people away from table salt due to the possibility that it contributes to high blood pressure and heart disease. Many people eat the healthier alternative, sea salt, which does not have added iodine.

Fluoridated water also contributes to iodine deficiency. Because of its structural similarity to iodine, fluoride competes with iodine for uptake by the thyroid gland and any other tissues that use iodine in your body. Bromide, a flame retardant used in bread doughs and sodas, does the same thing. Even when the average person consumes iodized salt, only 10% of the iodine is actually used by the body.[31]

Iodine deficiency creates more than just goiter. It can be linked to hypothyroidism, cretinism (stunted physical and mental growth), cognitive problems, neurological disorders, and breast disease. Iodine deficiency can also lead to irreversible damage in fetuses and newborns.

Are Nonorganic Foods Really Safe?

What do you put on your grass when the weeds are out of control? Roundup, of course! Roundup, or glyphosate, is the most commonly used herbicide among home gardeners. Farmers who plant genetically modified crops (GMOs) use glyphosate because these GMOs are genetically engineered to protect them from glyphosate's deadly effects. The idea is that the herbicide kills the weeds but not the crops. Weeds, however, are becoming more and more resistant to glyphosate, meaning more and more of the herbicide must be sprayed onto the crops.

The U.S. Environmental Protection Agency (EPA) considers glyphosate to be "practically nontoxic and not an irritant."[32] But is glyphosate really as safe as we have been told? Studies conducted by the chemical industry use much lower concentrations than what the average person is exposed to over long periods.[33]

Studies sponsored by the chemical industry on the toxicity of glyphosate are conducted on only a three-month basis. Three months is not enough time to accurately determine the effects of a chemical that consumers will eat over a lifetime. Only one study—wholly independent of the chemical industry—investigated the effects of GMO corn and soy treated with Roundup, fed to rats over the lifetime of the animals.[34] The study concluded that exposure to Roundup or even GMO foods alone increased the risk of breast tumors in females and increased the risk of kidney and liver damage in males. The overall lifespan of the animals decreased as well. The kicker? This damage did not appear until the **fourth** month of the study.

The combination of adjuvants and glyphosates found in Roundup is more toxic than just glyphosate alone.[35-37] In fact, one study found Roundup to be more 125x more toxic than glyphosate, leading the researchers to write, "Despite its relatively benign reputation, Roundup was among the most toxic herbicides and insecticides tested."[35]

Dr. Stephanie Seneff has conducted many studies on glyphosate, and what she's found is disturbing. Dr. Seneff theorized that glyphosate kills beneficial bacteria and believes there is a link between glyphosate and diseases such as Alzheimer's, celiac, autism, and even osteoporosis due to its ability to deplete the body's manganese levels.[38] Diagnoses of Alzheimer's and autism have skyrocketed in the last 20 years, coinciding with increased use of glyphosate on American crops.

According to Seneff, "From 1995 to 2010, the autism rates in first grade in the public school correlates almost perfectly with total glyphosate application on corn and soy crops over the previous four years (from age 2 to 6 for each child)."[38]

Another Myth: FDA-Approved = Safe

We've been conditioned to believe that the FDA seal of approval indicates total safety for our bodies. Wrong! We'll talk more about medication side effects in chapter 3 and throughout the book. Opioid painkillers are just one example of drugs that aren't as safe as we've been led to believe. Tragically, addiction to these drugs has become an epidemic. Worldwide, an estimated 26.4 million to 36 million people abuse opioids. Approximately 2.1 million Americans are addicted to these painkillers.[39]

This addiction comes with a steep price. More than 183,000 people in the U.S. have died from prescription opioid overdoses from 1999 to 2015.[40]

There are much safer and more effective ways to treat pain, such as changing the delivery method of certain painkillers via compounding (more on this in chapter 8). Pain relief can also be achieved by lowering inflammation through diet and lifestyle changes. We'll discuss these changes in detail throughout this book.

True Healthcare Reform

True healthcare reform can't be found in Washington, D.C. It can't be debated in the U.S. Senate or the House of Representatives, and no one can tell you that it is unconstitutional or unfair. That's because *true* healthcare reform starts and ends with **you.**

We're talking about a new type of healthcare reform where each and every person takes steps to understand what is truly best for them rather than what profit-hungry corporations declare to be healthy. This proactive approach involves lifestyle changes: optimizing your diet, exercise, and supplementation habits.

Properly prescribed pharmaceutical drugs have their place—for emergencies and when they are medically necessary.

The key to living a healthy life is to find a balance for everything, including sleep, diet, stress, and worry. Failure to be proactive regarding your health means the possibility of ending up on a gurney in a medical center, wishing you had cared more about wellness before. Many times, these tragedies happen sooner rather than later.

> *"There are no guarantees in the world when it comes to health. Misfortune can befall anyone. But if you consistently look both ways before crossing the street, you dramatically decrease your risk of being run over."*
>
> **— Dr. Chris Meletis**

In today's America, the health insurance industry guides the healthcare industry. But these insurance policies limit the types of treatment you can receive. Providers can only prescribe treatments deemed appropriate by the insurance industry. Sometimes insurance companies force patients to try less expensive (and less effective) drugs, and the treatment fails (more on this in the next chapter). Plus, insurance policies won't pay for nutritional supplements—despite the crucial role many supplements play in optimal health.

The U.S. is falling far behind much of the developed world regarding healthcare. We immerse ourselves in disease management instead of promoting wellness management. How broken is our system? Just look at the numbers: 17.1% of the American GDP is spent on healthcare per capita. This is more than other countries including France, Sweden, Germany, Canada, and Great Britain. Despite this gross overspending, the prevalence of degenerative and chronic diseases continues to rise.[41]

A study on people over the age of 50 found that Americans had higher rates of cancer, diabetes, and heart disease compared to their European counterparts. Nearly twice as many Americans exhibited heart disease. Compared to 16% of Americans, 11% of the European subjects had diabetes. Yanks had double the rate of arthritis and cancers as well.[42]

The United States continues to fall behind the rest of the world in the most important category of all: **health!**

Learning from History

In this consumer society, newer is better. The newest smartphone is surely an improvement over the last one. But what happens when that commercially hyped smartphone catches fire in your pocket? In our media-blizzard/information overload world, we often make assumptions and confer importance on what is new and novel instead of critically thinking about whether the latest medications or health inventions we see advertised are really better.

Before the advent of widespread antibiotic use in 1911, indigenous peoples from all over the world used foods, herbs, and other therapies that they had developed to support the innate capacity of the human body to heal and be well.

If you aren't pursuing an optimally healthy lifestyle, you dramatically increase the likelihood of needing medication or interventional and invasive care. When you're scoffed at for looking into "alternative" medicine, ask yourself what *alternative* medicine really is. Is it the medicine that has kept humanity alive since the dawn of time, or is it the modern drug and procedural-based medicine that has only been around for the last couple centuries?

Don't get me wrong, modern medicine has its place—and thank God for it. It saves lives every day. But we have to minimize our dependence on it by proactively seeking optimal health.

Be Skeptical

If a random person approached you in the grocery store parking lot to tell you how great a certain drug or food product was for you, would you treat that knowledge as the health gospel? Not likely, I'd guess.

What if that random person was a television news reporter out on a personal shopping trip? Would that change things? Perhaps they were a healthcare worker. Would your opinion on the veracity of their claims change? What would happen if the person sharing those "pearls of wisdom" with you was a pharmaceutical sales rep?

Once you get home, you turn on the TV and hear the same information on your nightly news program. Does that make the information truer than the statements spoken by the person in the parking lot? After all, they were likely just parroting back what they heard earlier on a similar report. Maybe. Who sponsored the programming? Could it be a pharmaceutical company? Perhaps it's a food product company advocating for the health benefits of their new product.

Here's the point: **Do your own independent research.** Use trusted sources, talk to the other members of your health-care triangle, and don't believe everything you hear. Assume everything is incentivized.

Reactive vs. Proactive: The Battle for True Health

Today's health-care professionals are not trained in proactive medicine. Instead, they are taught reactive medicine, where action is taken only **after** a problem or diagnosis occurs. Diabetes, heart disease, obesity, strokes, Alzheimer's, fibromyalgia, psoriasis, eczema, heartburn, autoimmune conditions, cancers, and other disorders and diseases are treated only after they have developed. The reaction is an attempt to correct a symptom or symptoms, and measuring effectiveness is often limited to lab results. This reaction is most often personified in the form of prescription drugs.

Proactive medicine, on the other hand, works to prevent the problem or diagnosis from ever occurring in the first place. This approach is all about creating an optimally healthy lifestyle, no matter the starting age or health status. My approach can be traced back to my **5 Pillars of Optimal Health,** which will be discussed in detail later in this book. Although following these Pillars can virtually wipe out many of these health conditions, the desired outcome would be to prevent them in the first place. Each of these diseases can be at least partially linked to lifestyle factors, meaning we play a role in bringing them upon ourselves due to our choices. Many of the choices you make each day are causing you to live a less than optimal life. Don't allow yourself to be caught in a perpetual subpar state.

Reactive medicine may slightly lengthen life expectancy, but are we getting what we bargained for? My personal vision of optimal life doesn't include nursing homes, prescription drugs, constant pain, lack of energy, no zeal for life, or the inability to recognize loved ones.

Here is a list of the most common complaints I hear on a daily basis:

- "I don't have any get-up-and-go, I lack energy."
- "After work, I have no energy left to enjoy life."
- "I have to lie down by mid-afternoon."
- "I can't sleep."
- "I can't relax."
- "I don't even want to have sex anymore."
- "I am always hurting."
- "I don't ever feel like exercising."
- "I just feel bad."
- "I'm stressed out."
- "I can't see/hear well anymore."

- "I can't lose weight."
- "My head hurts all the time."
- "I have headaches often."
- "I spend all my time at the doctor's office."
- "I don't enjoy life anymore."
- "When I eat, my stomach burns."
- "After meals, I bloat and have diarrhea."
- "I am always constipated."

I don't ever want to go down this path, and I don't want you to, either! The good news is, you don't have to. You can overcome these and other issues and feel awesome doing so. Learning to use proactive methods and following the 5 Pillars of Optimal Health to create healthy lifestyle changes will create positive reactions in your body—and typically, it will do so quickly.

To achieve these results, you must be willing to go against the grain. Remember that the typical American path leads to poor health. Open your mind to new ideas and ways of thinking. Be willing to educate yourself, and you will learn how God designed our bodies to thrive optimally.

Chris was shocked when he decided to join my OptiYou RX Wellness Summit, and we measured his lean muscle mass and body fat percentage. He had just completed a 12-week workout regimen with a group, and he was sure his numbers would be great.

Not so! Even though Chris could do amazing workouts he had not addressed his diet, supplements, or sleep. After just one week of following my OptiYou RX plan, he lost 13 pounds, and his joint pains disappeared.

In this book, I'm going to show you how to approach health differently than others. I'm going to share information with you that you likely won't hear elsewhere.

I want you to walk away from what you read here armed with the knowledge to take charge of your own health. My goal is for you to feel healthier and more energized than ever before.

Just like Janet did. Janet teaches yoga and is over 50 years old. She truly is one of the most amazing people my wife Beth and I have ever met. Janet broke her back but continues to heal and do things she was told she would never do again. Janet uses yoga to keep herself strong and flexible. She has spent countless hours rehabbing. Janet paid for nutritional training from a well-known teacher when she lived in Los Angeles. Then after attending my OptiYou RX Wellness Workshop, she decided to attend the OptiYou RX Wellness Summit. The changes she saw in just a few weeks were incredible. She is doing hand stands and other yoga poses she hasn't been able to do in years, plus her hands and fingers aren't swollen and sore anymore. She has dropped body fat despite eating more food than ever because she mistakenly believed, like many, that it is all about calories. She said, "Eating by the OptiYou RX plan is very liberating. I'm enjoying food again, and I feel like I'm 20 years old."

Chapter 1 OptiNotes

- Always be skeptical of health-related information. Verify sources, and do your own research! Only get your information from experts.
- You've been told myths about your health for your whole life, and these falsehoods are the reason you feel sick or fatigued.
- When it comes to health, Americans spend the most and get poor results.
- So-called "safe" foods can really be toxic. They profit the agriculture industry while stealing your well-being.
- Just because a drug is approved does not mean it is safe.
- When it comes to medicine, proactive > reactive. **The 5 Pillars of Optimal Health,** which you will learn about soon, will outline how to be proactive regarding health.
- If you suffer from many of the common issues we see in America today (low energy, low libido, headaches, can't lose weight, don't enjoy life, or just want to feel better), then you need this book.

- It is imperative to be skeptical and conduct your own research regarding foods, medications, and other chemicals that are put into your body. As we spend more and more on healthcare in America, we continue to get sicker. Don't be fooled by the massive amounts of money from within the system that cloud and obscure the facts. **You** have to take initiative to control your own health!

References

1. American Diabetes Association. http://www.diabetes.org/diabetes-basics/statistics/ Accessed November 25, 2016.

2. Menke A, et al. JAMA. 2015;314(10):1021-9.

3. Centers for Disease Control and Prevention. http://www.cdc.gov/diabetes/data/statistics/2014statisticsreport.html Accessed November 29, 2016.

4. Akhlaghi F, et al. Clin Pharmacokinet. 2016 Nov 10. [Epub ahead of print.]

5. D'Adamo E, Caprio S. Diabetes Care. 2011 May;34(Supplement 2):S161-5.

6. Mayo Clinic. http://www.mayoclinic.org/diseases-conditions/non-alcoholic-fatty-liver-disease/home/ovc-20211638 Accessed March 6, 2017.

7. Ogden CL, et al. JAMA. 2014 Feb 26;311(8):806-14.

8. Heidenreich PA, et al. Circulation. 2011;123:933-944.

9. UNC Carolina Population Center. http://demography.cpc.unc.edu/wp-content/uploads/2014/06/All-Cause-Mortality-and-Top-10_USA-e1402597040445.png Accessed November 25, 2016.

10. Centers for Disease Control. http://www.cdc.gov/heartdisease/facts.htm Accessed November 25, 2016.

11. S. Sinatra. The Great Cholesterol Myth. http://www.drsinatra.com/the-great-cholesterol-myth/ Accessed November 25, 2016.

12. Millán Núñez-Cortés J, et al. Am J Cardiovasc Drug. 2016 Nov 11. [Epub ahead of print.]

13. Rojas-Fernandez CH, Cameron JC. Ann Pharmacother. 2012 Apr;46(4):549-57.

14. Kritchevsky D, et al. Am J Physiol. 1954 Jul;178(1):30-2.

15. Lemmon RM, et al. Arch Biochem Biophys. 1954 Jul;51(1):161-9.

16. Kritchevsky D. J Atheroscler Res. 1964 Jan-Feb;4:103-5.

17. Thornley S, et al. Intern Med J. 2012 Oct;42 Suppl 5:46-58.

18. Mock K, et al. J Nutr Biochem. 2016 Sep 30;39:32-39.

19. Lin WT, et al. J Pediatr. 2016 Apr;171:90-6.e1.

20. Moose RM. Sugar a "diluting agent". JAMA 1944;125:738-9.

21. DiNicolantonio JJ, Berger A. Open Heart. 2016 Aug 2;3(2):e000469.

22. Lowndes J, et al. Nutrients. 2014 Mar;6(3):1128-44.

23. Yin L, et al. Ecotoxicol Environ Saf. 2016 Dec;134P1:213-25.

24. Food and Drug Administration. http://www.fda.gov/food/resourcesforyou/consumers/ucm110591.htm Accessed November 25, 2016.

25. Das K, Mondal NK. Environ Monit Assess. 2016 Apr;188(4):218.

26. Khan SA, et al. J Clin Diagn Res. 2015 Nov;9(11):ZC10-5.

27. Lv YG, et al. Biochem Biophys Res Commun. 2016 Oct 14;479(2):372-9.

28. Markel H. Am J Public Health 1987;77:219-29.

29. Hollowell JG, et al. J Clin Endocrinol Metab. 1998;83:3401-8.

30. Blackburn GL. Am J Clin Nutr. 2003;78:197-8.

31. Abraham GE. Original Internist 2004;11:29-38.

32. Bai SH, Ogbourne SM. Environ Sci Pollut Res Int. 2016 Oct;23(19):18988-9001.

33. Roy NM, et al. Environ Toxicol Pharmacol. 2016 Sep;46:292-300.

34. Séralini GE, et al. Environ Sci Eur. 2014;26:14.

35. Mesnage R, et al. Biomed Res Int. 2014.2014:179691.

36. Vincent K, Davidson C. Environ Toxicol Chem. 2015 Dec;34(12):2791-5.

37. Coalova I, et al. Toxicol In Vitro. 2014 Oct;28(7):1306-11.

38. Samsel A, Seneff S. Surg Neurol Int. 2015;6:45.

39. Volkow N. Senate Caucus on International Narcotics Control. May 14, 2014. https://www.drugabuse.gov/about-nida/legislative-activities/testimony-to-congress/2016/americas-addiction-to-opioids-heroin-prescription-drug-abuse

40. Centers for Disease Control and Prevention. https://www.cdc.gov/drugoverdose/data/overdose.html Accessed March 6, 2016.

41. The Commonwealth Fund. http://www.commonwealthfund.org/publications/issue-briefs/2015/oct/us-health-care-from-a-global-perspective Accessed November 25, 2016.

42. Thorpe KE, et al. Health Aff. (Millwood). 2007 Nov-Dec;26(6): w678-86.

CHAPTER 2

The "Medicine Mindset" and How It Is Destroying Your Health

"There are few areas of medical practice that are completely isolated from nutritional links or influences. Physicians must be prepared for the many situations when nutrition knowledge and clinical nutrition skills can improve the likelihood of optimal health outcomes."

— Martin Kohlmeier, M.D., Ph.D.,
University of North Carolina
Nutrition Research Institute

Modern America is vastly overmedicated. Here are some disturbing statistics from a society taking far too many prescription drugs:

- 4.2 billion prescriptions were written in the United States in 2011.[1]

- A study found that nearly 60% of adults 20 years and older had used at least one prescription drug in the past 30 days. Staggeringly, almost 15% had used 5 or more prescription drugs in the past 30 days.[2]

- According to the CDC, over 67% of doctor office visits result in a prescription being written, while more than 80% of hospital emergency room visits involve a prescription being written.[3]

- The average nursing home resident takes 7 to 8 prescription drugs. Roughly one-third of nursing home residents take 9 or more medications.[4, 5]

- Approximately 128,000 people die every year from properly pre-scribed prescription drugs (this means no mistakes leading to complications were made by any involved parties). That places prescription drugs squarely as the 4th leading cause of death in the U.S., tied with stroke.

- 60,000 people died as a result of taking the drug Vioxx before it was taken off the market. This was just one of many prescription drugs approved and later removed due to harmful side effects.[6]

These statistics are shocking. As a traditionally-trained pharmacist, I now understand that this over-reliance on drugs is what all healthcare professionals are taught by their university programs. Both medical and pharmacy schools emphasize reacting to diagnoses with a drug regimen.

When I decided to attend pharmacy school, I wanted to help people get well and stay well. The desire to have that ability on a daily basis is what motivated me to enter the health-care field in the first place. That's why I believe the medical education system needs an overhaul. It's time to step back and evaluate the benefits of teaching proactive healthy alternatives as the first line of treatment rather than continuing to promote reactive medicine and prescription drugs.

Take a look at these statistics:

- Only 1 in 4 physicians feel they receive adequate training to counsel patients on diet or physical activity.[7]
- Medical students in the U.S. receive an average of just 24 hours of nutrition instruction during medical school.[8]
- 88% of medical school instructors would like additional nutrition education at their universities.[8]

Is it any wonder that many doctors don't realize that nutrition can be used to promote health?

A Biased Education

When I was working for Eckerd Drugs, it became obvious that none of my regular customers were getting well. Many actually saw their health worsen, with new complications arising and new drugs often added simply to maintain their current unhealthy status.

The pharmaceutical industry is a powerful and influential entity in modern America. Drug companies (collectively known as Big Pharma) have money and resources at their disposal that I can only dream of. The top 11 global pharmaceutical companies raked in *$85 billion* in net profits in 2012.[9] Big Pharma subsidizes, donates, and in many cases *controls* the agendas taught in pharmacy and other medical programs throughout American colleges.

Did you know that the word "doctor" means "teacher"? The idea is that the doctors should educate patients on how to become healthy.

That was the case in many medical schools prior to the early 1900s, when two families decided to take control of medical school agendas. In 1910, many medical schools were shut down, especially those teaching natural and homeopathic health. This was a result of The Flexner Report (also known as Carnegie Foundation Bulletin Number Four), which called for medical schools to adhere strictly to the author's definition of "modern" medicine or be shut down. This led to the forced closing of many schools that taught chiropractic, naturopathic, and homeopathic therapies.

The schools that survived were forced to place donors on their board of directors, and the **pharmaceutical monopoly** began. These medical schools were then obligated to teach reactive medicine—and nothing else. If the schools taught anything beyond the required pharmaceutical drug treatment doctrine, their funding would be cut off.

By 1925, more than 10,000 herbalists were out of business as a result of the Flexner doctrine. By 1950, every single homeopathic school had been shuttered. Any professional who did not graduate from a Flexner-approved medical school was shunned by the industry. Natural treatments were discouraged and ridiculed. The doctrine of heavy pharmaceutical use took hold and has grown at an alarming degree. Today, the U.S. consists of less than 5% of the world's population yet consumes over 70% of the world's pain medication prescription drugs. The financial costs are high for millions of Americans, but the health costs are steeper.

Hippocrates, the celebrated "Father of Modern Medicine," told us to "Let food be thy medicine." The modern medical establishment's ignorance on this front is at least partly responsible for the deteriorating quality of health care in America. According to a report published in the *Journal of the American Medical Association (JAMA),* death caused by the medical system is ranked third on a list of leading mortality causes, behind only heart disease and cancer.[10] Are we getting our money's worth? Or is the American medical industry more concerned with income gains than your health? **Stop being a victim of the "profit over patient" system!**

Most doctors surveyed today list pharmaceutical reps and articles sponsored by pharmaceutical industries as their main source of information after graduation. It only makes sense that the pharmaceutical companies responsible for much of their medical school training continue to provide information to these doctors after the fact. And let's face it: after all the time, money, and hard work invested in grueling years of medical schooling, it must be difficult for medical professionals to change the ideas, philosophies, and methods that were repeatedly pounded into their heads regarding the best treatment. Healthcare providers can't teach what they aren't taught and in many cases never have the opportunity to learn. This is why I had to go out and further my education after pharmacy school.

The Modern Healthcare System Doesn't Have Your Best Interests at Heart

The healthcare system in America is programmed to react with drugs to complaints, conditions, and diseases. Patients are no different; marketing and precedent have programmed us to expect, want, ask about, and in many cases, demand a drug for our illnesses or conditions. The pharmaceutical industry spends more money each year on marketing their drugs than they do on research to make sure the drugs are safe. This has led to the current American thought that drugs are the first and only treatment option.[26]

From infancy, we are taught by our parents and caretakers to always follow the advice of our doctors. We trust healthcare professionals to do what is best for us.

Unfortunately, other factors at play mean the healthcare system is not always operating exclusively in our favor. Insurance companies can make deals wherein pharmaceutical companies pay them a reimbursement fee every time a certain drug is dispensed to one of their clients. This is why pharmacies often call physicians' offices to ask if it's ok to use an alternative drug to what the doctor wrote. The insurance company wants the kickback payment from the drug company despite what the doctor prescribed, so they try to force the pharmacy to fill that, instead. Sometimes the drug the insurance company mandates is less expensive, but it may not necessarily be a better treatment.

Additionally, insurance companies have cut healthcare reimbursement rates drastically for doctors, pharmacists, and all healthcare providers. Now the volume of patients that a doctor needs to see or the number of prescriptions that a pharmacy needs to fill daily in order to stay in business makes it hard to spend time with patients and customers, much less spending time doing real research on which treatments are best.

The result? For the most common diseases and conditions today, the go-to treatments are almost exclusively prescription and over-the-counter drugs. These drugs are just Band-Aids and don't really fix the conditions that created the original problem. It's the equivalent of putting a small bandage on a gash to slow the bleeding but never healing the cut. This is the treatment administered over and over and over for the most prevalent diseases in America today. We use side effect-laden drugs to mask symptoms and never really address the underlying problem, so the patient never really gets better. We aren't addressing the root cause of our health problems; this is why the drugs are not working!

Drugs Are Making You Sicker

Not only are pharmaceutical drugs not working, they're making our health problems worse. As mentioned earlier, diabetes is now an American epidemic, but the proliferation of diabetes drugs isn't working for kids or adults. The Action to Control Cardiovascular Risk in Diabetes (ACCORD) trials actually showed that diabetics treated more aggressively with conventional medicine died sooner![11] This is because of the refusal to treat diabetes properly. Conventional medicine approaches it as a disease of too little insulin, but in fact, insulin resistance is the culprit—in some cases, there is already too much insulin! The idea of using drugs that increase insulin production and/or insulin shots is counter-productive and comes with a long list of side effects.

Heart disease is still treated as a problem of excess cholesterol despite the fact that **75%** of people hospitalized for a heart attack have perfectly **normal** cholesterol levels.[12] The standard of care is to prescribe a drug to lower cholesterol, typically from a class of drugs known as *statins*. Statin drugs have harmful side effects and do not address the real culprits of heart disease—not to mention their exorbitant cost.

To make matters worse, a majority of diabetics are prescribed statin drugs *despite* the fact that statins have been shown to *increase* incidences of diabetes. Once again, this can be traced back to what doctors are taught in medical school: that diabetics and heart-disease patients, according to the standard of care, should be prescribed cholesterol-lowering drugs. Today, almost anyone with even slightly elevated or borderline cholesterol levels are given statin drugs.[27]

Many people who have heart disease and/or diabetes are also prescribed drugs to treat high blood pressure. These drugs don't address the real causes of high blood pressure and only mask the numbers. Furthermore, according to the American Heart Association (AHA), drugs designed to lower blood pressure are becoming less and less effective.[13] But rather than recommend lifestyle changes to increase effectiveness, the AHA claims that people with high blood pressure are sicker to begin with and need additional drugs and higher doses to control their hypertension.[13,14]

A review published in the *Cochrane Database of Systematic Reviews* found that people with mild hypertension received no benefit from blood pressure-lowering drugs. Compared with a placebo, the antihypertensive drugs did not reduce either total mortality, coronary heart disease, strokes, or total cardiovascular events.[15]

Antihypertensive medications are also accompanied by a laundry list of side effects. In fact, 9% of the *Cochrane* review subjects had to drop out of the study due to adverse side effects from the drugs.[15]

Controlling high blood pressure is critically important, and you should not ignore this problem. But your goal should be to treat the cause, not the symptom, and create the best outcome.

Even when the conventional medical establishment recommends lifestyle changes to treat disease, their suggestions are often incorrect. Heart patients and diabetics are typically prescribed a low-fat diet, which has virtually no positive effects on the patients' health. Low-fat diets don't even improve the important cholesterol factors, such as lowering triglycerides.

Challenging the Status Quo

The conventional medical establishment's views are no different with cancer. 1 in 3 Americans will develop cancer in their lifetime. The standard treatments, as you may have guessed, are not addressing the real problems. Instead of strengthening the body and fueling its ability to fight using its powerful immune system, many cancer treatments destroy our immunity.

Our immune system is the body's God-given way to fight many diseases, especially in the case of cancer. The standard treatments of chemotherapy and radiation are actually carcinogenic, which means they are known to **cause** cancer. This is one reason why someone treated for cancer is often pronounced "cancer-free" only to develop another or the same type of cancer later. Unfortunately, their immune system is weakened from the first round of treatments, and their body has more difficulty overcoming this second cancer.

I'm not saying that people diagnosed with cancer should not use conventional treatments. But they should be fully informed about both the myriad side effects **and** about alternative methods to try and overcome this terrible disease. Big Pharma and our medical system have dictated a standard of treatment that doctors must follow, even if they do not believe it is the only choice for patients.

Scientists from the McGill Cancer Center conducted polls and questionnaires of 118 doctors who were cancer experts and found that 3 out of 4 would not use chemotherapy if they had cancer.[16] Why? Because of the damaging consequences to the entire body and the immune system.

Not only is mainstream cancer treatment flawed, but cancer diagnostic processes are also harmful. Mammograms expose women to radiation and often yield false positives. Thermograms are safer and more effective at screening for breast cancer. Why then aren't women educated about and offered thermograms? Because mammograms are big business, and doctors are taught in medical school that they are the only option.

An imbalance in estrogen and progesterone levels contributes to many cancers, especially in females. Prescription drugs in the form of birth control pills, common menopause drugs, and other medications are often to blame for imbalances in these hormone levels. Once these cancers are diagnosed, the patients are prescribed additional drugs to fight the tumors. Many of these hormone-related cancers can be prevented and even treated with compounded bioidentical hormones and lifestyle changes.

Our healthcare system waits until cancer diagnosis to take action instead of employing methods that are proven to help prevent cancer development in the first place. This is just another instance of our healthcare system being reactive instead of proactive.

Getting to the Root Cause of Your Health Problems

As I watched my customers continue to take drugs and not get any better, I decided a change had to be made. I couldn't stand around and watch people's health deteriorate when I knew I could help, given the opportunity. This shaped the vision for my independent pharmacy, where I could spend time talking to people and assisting them with their health conditions. Later in the book, you will learn about the OptiYou RX Program that can help you make lifestyle changes to promote a vibrant and healthy lifestyle with less reliance on drugs.

It's not that I want you to avoid drugs completely. There is a time and place for pharmaceuticals. People with hypertension need antihypertensive medications, for example. But by implementing proper lifestyle changes, we can stabilize blood pressure and help clients safely discontinue these medications under the guidance of their doctor.

Likewise, antibiotics for infections, insulin for diabetics, epinephrine for anaphylactic shock, inhalers for asthma, and antidepressant drugs are all necessary until the cause behind the condition can be pinpointed and resolved.

But many times drugs truly **aren't** needed. Even the CDC admits that antibiotics are prescribed for 80% of bronchitis cases. The problem? Antibiotics aren't even recommended for bronchitis in the first place.[17]

This errant overprescribing only encourages more widespread antibiotic resistance. At least 2 million Americans develop serious antibiotic-resistant infections each year.[18] At least 23,000 people die annually as a direct result of antibiotic resistance.

When the Treatment Is Worse Than the Disease

Next time a TV commercial for a pharmaceutical drug comes on, turn up the volume and listen to the announcer race through the ridiculous list of side effects. Kidney failure, liver failure, heart failure, increased risk of cancer, and **sudden death** are just some of the possible side effects mentioned. My goal in writing this book is to make sure you think about the effects these drugs have on your body and to better educate you about natural alternatives like lifestyle changes that can often correct or improve our health problems with **only** positive side effects.

The average pharmaceutical drug lists 69 side effects on its package insert. That's what drug companies **admit** to. A study from the University of Stanford School of Medicine found that the average prescription drug had 329 **additional** side effects not listed by the manufacturers.[19] That adds up to a staggering **398** side effects for just one prescription drug, on average. If you take more than one prescription drug, you risk 398 potential side effects from each drug, plus countless drug interaction effects.

That number should shock you. It sure shocked me, and it was just another reason why I became wary of prescription drugs as a first resort in treatments. Sadly, very few even know that many of these side effects exist. Drug companies do not inform healthcare professionals about these numerous adverse reactions. Because drug companies impact health education so significantly, university students in the healthcare field are not educated about this, either.

People over the age of 65 should not take certain medications at all. *Beers Criteria for Potentially Inappropriate Medication Use in the Elderly* recognizes nearly 50 medications and pharmaceutical drug classes that can harm senior patients.[20] Many of these drugs are considered by *Beers* to cause not just mild side effects but severe adverse outcomes.

Patients pay the price for healthcare providers being unfamiliar with all the side effects of drugs—and with 398 on average, how could they be? Take Joe for example. Joe was a very active person in his late 60s. He walked every morning, maintained an ideal weight, and had normal cholesterol and blood pressure levels. Based on his lab results and routine checkups, Joe was the picture of health. Joe followed the low-fat diet his doctor recommended.

One morning on his daily walk, Joe began having chest pains and had to stop at a stranger's house and ask them to call 911. An ambulance rushed Joe to the hospital, where he was diagnosed with a heart attack resulting from blockages in several arteries in and around his heart.

After open-heart surgery, Joe was sent home with a multitude of prescription drugs—the ones typically prescribed after a heart attack. One of these drugs was a commonly prescribed statin, ostensibly to lower Joe's cholesterol even though his levels were normal. He was also given a beta blocker medication to help control his heart rate. Joe was advised to continue following a low-fat, low-cholesterol diet and continue exercising.

After just a few days of home recovery, Joe began walking daily again. He was recuperating to his pre-heart attack routine but noticed a great deal of leg pain and overall fatigue. The problems worsened and became noticeable even when he wasn't exercising. The leg pain was especially prominent at night, hindering his sleep.

Joe asked his doctor and pharmacist about his symptoms. He was told they were normal, and it would take time to get his strength and endurance back. The doctor prescribed Joe a sleeping pill from the benzodiazepine class of drugs to help with his difficulty sleeping.

The drug helped Joe sleep better for a while, but the fatigue and leg pain continued. It wasn't long before his sleeping became fitful again. He developed leg cramps and was diagnosed with restless leg syndrome. This diagnosis led to another prescription drug treatment, which helped temporarily but then stopped working just like the others he was still taking.

Joe had quickly gone from seemingly perfect health to suffering from fatigue, muscle pain, restless legs, and poor sleep. What could be the cause of these issues? Neither his doctor--the top cardiologist in his area--nor his pharmacist could solve his problems.

Sadly, Joe's medication regimen was certainly contributing to—if not causing—his adverse symptoms, and his healthcare team was unable to identify the problem. Of course, medications were swapped and dosages adjusted, but Joe was unable to overcome these problems for the rest of his life.

Leg pain, muscle pain, and fatigue are all known side effects of statin drugs. These drugs block the production of coenzyme Q10—one-third of the energy source for every cell in our bodies, especially our muscle cells. This is why statins have muscle-related side effects. The beta blocker Joe was taking can cause fatigue and cramping. The benzodiazepine prevented him from reaching a restorative sleep state, further contributing to his fatigue. Ironically, this class of drugs reduces levels of melatonin, the hormone produced to help foster good sleep.[28, 29]

Joe is the perfect example of the cascade of side effects that prescription drugs can cause. Neither his cardiologist nor his pharmacist recognized the results.

I am ashamed to admit that I was Joe's pharmacist. At the time, I didn't know that statins depleted CoQ10 or that the side effects from all these drugs were causing Joe's problems. These side effects weren't emphasized in pharmacy school, and this was before I sought additional education in metabolic and nutritional medicine. Cardiologists aren't taught about the potential dangers of these side effects, either; that's why many of them ask why I recommend CoQ10 supplements for my customers who are on statin drugs.

Prescribing CoQ10 to patients on statin drugs should be standard protocol in the U.S. as it is in most European countries. Many of Joe's side effects could have been prevented with the addition of a professionally-formulated, pharmaceutical-grade CoQ10 supplement. Joe could have further benefited from a good magnesium supplement to combat his fatigue, heart condition, restless legs, and sleep problems.

Of course, statins aren't the only medications with side effects. Consider the potential side effects of drugs prescribed for attention deficit disorder and attention deficit hyperactive disorder. Many are amphetamine-type drugs that wreak havoc on the body's adrenal glands, heart, blood pressure regulation, and appetite control. They can also cause growth issues in children.[21] Despite all this, these ADD and ADHD drugs are dispensed to millions of children every day.

Are Over-the-Counter Drugs Safe?

In many cases, over-the-counter (OTC) drugs are no safer than their prescription counterparts. Many are similar versions of prescription drugs such as heartburn and acid reflux drugs known as proton pump inhibitors (PPIs). Many of these drugs are available with or without a prescription. They can be purchased just about anywhere, including gas stations or convenience stores, without the advice of a health-care professional.

These drugs work by blocking the acid production of the stomach's proton pump. Although this method often reduces acid reflux or heartburn symptoms, the true problem is typically a lack of enzymes and/or too **little** stomach acid production.

PPI drugs will **never** fix the underlying issue. Instead of improving your health, they are likely to make it worse. PPIs are known to cause or contribute to hip fractures, poorer nutrient digestion and utilization, and increased risk of heart failure and death in people with coronary artery disease, dementia, and kidney disease.[22-25]

PPIs also lower levels of calcium, magnesium, and vitamin B12. More on this in the next chapter.

Treat the Cause, Not the Symptoms

Our healthcare system's problem is its increased focus on treating symptoms instead of causes.

Instead of prescribing PPIs, we should address one of the underlying causes of acid reflux: too little good bacteria or probiotics and enzymes in the digestive system. Supplementing with high-quality probiotic and digestive enzyme formulas can improve or completely stop heartburn and acid reflux symptoms. Taking proper probiotics and digestive enzymes usually yields positive results within 2 to 3 days. Many people on this regimen report that their reflux and heartburn symptoms disappear. That's because this approach fixes the cause and improves the digestive system's ability to work properly as well as enhances the body's immune system.

Callie's story is one you should pay close attention to. She is a nurse and suffered for over 20 years. In her own words:

> As I entered nursing school, my stomach problems began. My stomach hurt every day. I did everything the doctors asked, including different drugs and tests. Nothing ever seemed to help, and it was so discouraging.
>
> As time passed, I learned to live with the daily stomach pain but continued to see my health go downhill. Over the 20-plus-year

period before I met Billy and began the OptiYou RX Program, I was diagnosed with almost everything you can imagine: eosinophilic esophagitis (EoE), candida, fibromyalgia, endometriosis, obesity, gastroesophageal reflux disease, pre-diabetes, and more. But the crazy thing was, nothing I or the doctors tried helped, and my quality of life with daily pain was terrible.

At the OptiYou RX Wellness Workshop, I started crying because I couldn't believe that at 39 years old, I had allowed myself to become this sick. And even worse, I work in the medical profession and still could not get any help. My health was a burden, not only to me but to my husband and children. But I remember Billy saying that this was a new beginning, and the insanity of trying things that didn't work for over 20 years would come to an end if I would listen and become the chief executive officer (CEO) of my own health.

After 2 to 3 weeks of the OptiYou RX Program, my stomach pain disappeared and never returned. I began to lose fat, felt amazing energy, and began working out at Billy's CrossFit gym. I discontinued all my prescription medications and felt better than I had in over 20 years.

I set a goal to be healthy by 40, and I am glad to say that by the time my birthday rolled around, I had lost 55 pounds of fat while gaining 2 pounds of muscle and dropped my body fat percentage from 50 percent to 35 percent. Plus, I feel great.

My husband lost fat and was able to discontinue his 4 blood pressure prescription medications also. I even saw positive changes in my kids' bodies and attitudes.

I thank Billy and the entire OptiYou RX team for all the life-changing information, support, consultations, and encouragement to help me and my family achieve optimal health, wellness, and fitness.

God designed our bodies to work as amazing machines, capable of functioning at a high level, free from disease when given what they need and not what they don't. Throughout this book, I will explain what your body needs to feel healthy, vibrant, and free from disease. I'll show you how to fix problems instead of just masking symptoms.

Select Side Effects of Some Common Drugs	
Atenolol (blood pressure)	<ul><li>constipation, indigestion</li><li>dizziness, faintness</li><li>dry mouth</li><li>impotence</li><li>cold extremities (hands and feet)</li><li>confusion</li><li>depression</li><li>insomnia, nightmares</li></ul>
Lisinopril [Prinivil and Zestril] (blood pressure)	<ul><li>cough</li><li>dizziness, drowsiness, headache</li><li>depressed mood</li><li>nausea, vomiting, diarrhea, upset stomach</li><li>mild skin itching, rash</li><li>angioedema (potentially dangerous swelling of the face or throat)</li></ul>
Paxil, Prozac, Zoloft, Celexa, Lexapro, Viibryd (selective serotonin reuptake inhibitors as antidepressants)	<ul><li>drowsiness</li><li>nausea</li><li>dry mouth</li><li>insomnia</li><li>diarrhea</li><li>nervousness, agitation, restlessness</li><li>dizziness</li><li>reduced sexual desire, difficulty reaching orgasm, erectile dysfunction</li></ul>

Prilosec, Yosprala, Prevacid, Dexilant, Aciphex, Nexium, Protonix (proton pump inhibitors for acid reflux and heartburn)	• weakened bones • poor digestion and utilization of foods • increased risk of heart disease, high blood pressure, kidney disease • headache • nausea • diarrhea • abdominal pain • fatigue • dizziness • rash • itching • flatulence • constipation • anxiety • depression • myopathies including rhabdomyolysis (rapid breakdown of skeletal muscle which can lead to kidney failure)
Fosamax, Zometa, Reclast, Boniva, Atelvia, Actonel, Binosto, Skelid, Aclasta (bisphosphonates for osteoporosis)	• high temperature (fever) and flu-like symptoms (more common when given by drip) • low calcium levels • bone and joint pain • constipation or diarrhea • tiredness • sick feeling • kidney damage • osteonecrosis of the jaw • blocking of bone turnover

Lipitor, Crestor, Mevacor, Pravachol, Livalo (statin drugs for cholesterol)	• headaches • insomnia • flushing of skin • muscle aches, tenderness, weakness (myalgia) • drowsiness • dizziness • nausea, vomiting • abdominal cramping, pain
Plavix (blood thinner)	• itching • eczema • rash • head pain, joint pain • bruising • diarrhea • fever • skin redness • taste problems • nosebleed • bloody or tarry stool • blood in urine • coughing up blood • vomiting that looks like coffee grounds • crushing heavy chest pain that spreads to arm, shoulder, jaw • sudden numbness or weakness, especially on one side of the body • sudden headache • confusion

	<ul><li>vision problems, speech problems, balance problems</li><li>weakness</li><li>jaundice (pale skin, yellowing of skin or eyes)</li><li>purple or red pinpoint spots under skin</li><li>unusual bleeding in mouth, vagina, rectum</li></ul>

Chapter 2 OptiNotes

- People are taking far too many drugs. Why are so many prescribed?
- Prescriptions can kill, even when used properly.
- American healthcare is reactive instead of proactive and preventative.
- The pharmaceutical industry sways legislation and agendas with money and influence.
- Pharmaceutical companies aren't in the business of wellness; their goal is continual prescriptions that make them rich.
- Insurance companies may be reimbursed a specified amount each time a particular drug is dispensed for a patient.
- Drugs can often make us sicker, not healthier.
- Be informed and question standard procedures that keep making people sicker.
- There is a time and place for drugs. Working with the right pharmacist and doctor can help you understand which medications may be right for you.
- Some medications have side effects so bad that they are worse than the condition they are supposed to treat.

- Healthcare professionals are taught lots about the benefits of medications but never about all the side effects. Knowing side-effect information is crucial for a patient's health. Many patient complaints are caused by their medications.

- The most effective way to heal the body is to fix what is causing the problem rather than just treating the symptoms.

References

1. Lindsley CW. ACS Chemical Neuroscience. 2012;3(8):630.

2. Kantor ED, et al.JAMA. 2015;314(17):1818-30.

3. Centers for Disease Control. http://www.cdc.gov/nchs/fastats/drug-use-therapeutic.htm Accessed December 5, 2016.

4. Doshi JA, et al. J Am Geriatr Soc. 2005 Mar;53(3):438-43.

5. Light DW. Harvard University Center for Ethics. http://ethics.harvard.edu/blog/new-prescription-drugs-major-health-risk-few-offsetting-advantages Accessed December 5, 2016.

6. http://articles.mercola.com/sites/articles/archive/2012/05/14/mercks-adhd-drugs-unsafe.aspx. Accessed December 5, 2016.

7. Adams et al. and Howe et al. Centers for Disease Control and Prevention & National Center for Health Statistics. 2010.

8. Darer JD, et al. Acad Med. 2004 Jun;79(6):541-8.

9. Alternet.http://www.alternet.org/11-major-drug-companies-raked-85-billion-last-year-and-left-many-die-who-couldnt-buy-their-pricey. Accessed December 5, 2016.

10. Starfield B. JAMA. 2000 Jul 26;284(4):483-5.

11. Siraj ES, et al. Diabetes Care. 2015 Nov;38(11):2000-8.

12. UCLA press release. http://newsroom.ucla.edu/releases/majority-of-hospitalized-heart-75668 Accessed December 5, 2016.

13. New York Times. http://www.nytimes.com/2008/06/24/health/research/24bloo.html Accessed December 5, 2016.

14. Calhoun DA, et al. Hypertension. 2008;51:1403-19.

15. Diao D, et al. Cochrane Database Syst Rev. 2012 Aug 15;(8):CD006742.

16. Natural News. http://www.naturalnews.com/036054_chemotherapy_physicians_toxicity.html Accessed December 5, 2016.

17. Association of Missouri Nurse Practitioners. https://amnp.enpnetwork.com/nurse-practitioner-news/122941-cdc-antibiotics-for-bronchitis-not-needed-but-given-80-of-time Accessed December 5, 2016.

18. Centers for Disease Control. http://www.cdc.gov/drugresistance/threat-report-2013/ Accessed December 5, 2016.

19. Stanford Medicine. https://med.stanford.edu/news/all-news/2012/03/scientists-discover-multitude-of-drug-side-effects-interactions-using-new-computer-algorithm.html Accessed December 5, 2016.

20. Fick DM, et al. Arch Intern Med. 2003;163(22):2716-24.

21. Swanson JM, et al. J Child Psychol Psychiatr. 2017 Mar 10. [Epub ahead of print.] doi:10.1111/jcpp.12684

22. Adams AL, et al. Ann Epidemiol. 2014 Apr;24(4):286-90.

23. Pello Lázaro AM, et al. PLoS One. 2017 Jan 19;12(1):e0169826.

24. Tai SY, et al. PLoS One. 2017 Feb 15;12(2):e0171006.

25. Xie Y, et al. Kidney Int. 2017 Feb 20. [Epub ahead of print.] doi: 10.1016/j.kint.2016.12.021.

26. https://www.washingtonpost.com/news/wonk/wp/2015/02/11/big-pharmaceutical-companies-are-spending-far-more-on-marketing-than-research/?utm_term=.6c583ff4a777

27. https://www.ncbi.nlm.nih.gov/pubmed/28667223

28. https://www.ncbi.nlm.nih.gov/pubmed/27294339

29. https://www.ncbi.nlm.nih.gov/pmc/articles/PMC5104627/

CHAPTER 3

Is Your Medicine Cabinet Starving You of Crucial Nutrients?

I mentioned earlier that over 100,000 people die from properly pre-scribed prescription drugs every year. It should come as no surprise, then, that prescription and OTC drugs come with a fairly long list of potential side effects. While it's true that drugs often have sufficient power to change the chemistry of your body in a way that can treat disease, it is also true that they have sufficient power to negatively disrupt the balance of your body chemistry.

Let's take a look at some statistics[1] that illustrate why you should be concerned about the side effects of medications you may take and why you should always talk to your primary care physician and 21st Century Pharmacist to find out about drug-nutrient and drug-to-drug interactions.

- There is a 1-in-5 chance that a drug will cause a serious reaction after it has already been approved. This is one reason that knowl-edgeable healthcare providers and experts suggest trying an older and more established medication until new drugs have been on the market for five years. Exceptions are made for patients who exhibit an allergy to the established medications, patients who haven't responded to it, or other concerns.

- 840,000 hospitalized patients experience serious adverse reactions, for a total of 2.74 million serious adverse drug reactions per year.

- Over 1.9 million hospitalizations occur each year from properly prescribed drugs (this does not include misprescribed drugs, over-dosing, or self-prescribing).

- 128,000 people die from drugs prescribed to them each year.

- Death from prescribed drugs is the 4th leading cause of death in the U.S., tied with stroke.

- 170 million Americans take a prescription drug. 80% of drugs taken are generic.

Isaac Newton theorized a principle that most of us learned in high school science. Although this concept does not directly speak to nutrient deficiencies caused by drugs, it captures the spirit of the issue:

"For every action, there is an equal and opposite reaction."

— Newton's Third Law

Newton may not have been thinking about the impact of drugs within the human body, but it does make sense that if a medication has the potential for positive impact, it could also have potential for negative impact, either directly or in a secondary (less direct) pathway.

This is common sense. If you nudge or shove a biochemical pathway in your body, it results in a ripple effect. The intent of a medication can meet the therapeutic expectation or overshoot or fall short. Because the trillions of cells that comprise your body work in unison, the influence of a medication can often impact other tissues and parts of the body in addition to the intended target.

One of the most disturbing effects of pharmaceutical drugs is their ability to cause nutrient deficiencies or affect the way nutrients are used by the body. More than 100 medications reduce magnesium levels, which the average American is **already** deficient in. The extent to which a drug impacts nutrient bioavailability can depend on factors such as individual biochemical patterns and the duration of the drug therapy. Having low levels of specific nutrients not only damages your health, it can **worsen** the side effects of certain drugs.

These are often reflections of what I describe as the law of unintended consequences.

Drugs and nutrients interact in five ways:

1. Some drugs directly lower nutrient absorption.
2. Some drugs alter the effects of nutrients within the body.
3. Some drugs lead to increased loss of nutrients from the body.
4. Some drugs are much more toxic due to altered nutrient bioavailability in genetically susceptible individuals.
5. Low nutrient levels may increase the likelihood and severity of drug side effects.

There are even some instances where a particular botanical, vitamin, or dietary supplement can interfere with the effects of a drug.

It's critical that you also find out about drug-drug interactions. These take place when one drug changes the effects of another medicine, possibly causing more harm. The types of medicines in which these reactions are likely to occur include:[2]

- highly protein bound medicines such as aspirins and sulfonamides
- medicines that change the way your body metabolizes the drug such as the anti-epileptic drug phenytoin, the nerve pain and seizure medicine carbamazepine, and the antibiotic rifampicin
- medicines that block drug metabolism such as the antifungals cimetidine, metronidazole, and triazole.

These certainly aren't the only drugs that can interact with other medicines. There is potential for plenty of other harmful interplay between medications.

A 21st Century Pharmacist will help you discover which medicines cause nutrient deficiencies and which nutrients interact with drugs.

That's why it's so important to establish a single pharmacy home and know your pharmacist well. This way, the pharmacist can know your health issues and monitor all the medications you take.

In this chapter, I'll discuss just a handful of the thousands of nutrient depletions, interactions, and considerations that occur when you take a pharmaceutical drug. My goal in writing this chapter is to emphasize the importance of asking your healthcare professionals about these negative effects before taking the drug. This way, you can correct nutrient deficiencies caused by the drug and avoid using any other pharmaceuticals that react in a damaging way with the medication.

Drugs That Directly Lower Nutrient Absorption

Antibiotics

Your gastrointestinal (GI) tract is highly populated with microbes (good and bad bacteria) known as microbiota. By virtue of their ability to alter the microbiota, antibiotics can deplete levels of crucial vitamins. For example, the antibiotics cephalosporin, fluoroquinolone, isoniazid, macrolide, penicillin, sulfonamide, tetracyclines, and trimethoprim/sulfamethoxazole interfere with the liver circulation of folate and stop it from being reabsorbed.[3] These antibiotics may also lower the production of folate.[3] The antibiotic trimethoprim blocks folate's conversion into its active form.[4]

Metformin (Glucophage)

The anti-diabetes drug metformin interferes with the absorption of vitamin B12 and possibly folate.[5] According to the Glucophage package insert, controlled clinical trials of metformin showed that the drug caused a decline of vitamin B12 levels in approximately 7% of people taking it. However, some studies have reported that an average of 10% to 30% of patients taking metformin suffered from vitamin B12 deficiency due to decreased absorption of the vitamin.[6,7]

Don't take vitamin B12 deficiency lightly. This vitamin is crucial to many aspects of your health. Deficiency leads to peripheral neuropathy and painful nerve damage in type 2 diabetic patients.[5] Vitamin B12 deficiency is also linked to tinnitus (ringing in the ears),[8] a decline in cognitive function[9] and cardiovascular problems.[10,11] Of course, increase in risk of neuropathy leads to increased risk of being medicated for neuropathy, leading to more potential interactions. It's a vicious cycle.

The Glucophage package insert suggests measuring vitamin B12 levels every two to three years in patients who don't get enough B12 in their diet or who don't absorb it well. Supplementation with vitamin B12 can correct the metformin-caused deficiency. Calcium supplementation is also effective because it is involved in the vitamin B12 absorption process in the small intestine.[7]

Proton Pump Inhibitors

PPIs include lansoprazole (Prevacid), omeprazole (Losec, Prilosec), rabeprazole (Aciphex), and pantoprazole (Pantoloc, Protonix). These acid reflux drugs have the ability to block the absorption of magnesium, calcium, and vitamin B12.[12,13,14] Low magnesium can have disastrous effects on your neuromuscular, central nervous, and cardiovascular systems. Low magnesium can cause muscle spasms known as tetany, convulsions, slowed heart function (bradycardia), low blood pressure (hypotension), and even death. There have been reports of people becoming critically ill due to magnesium deficiency caused by PPIs.[15]

It's best to have your doctor test your red blood cell magnesium rather than your blood levels of magnesium. Blood levels of magnesium can sometimes appear normal even as the magnesium is not being delivered into the blood cells.

Nutrient deficiencies that arise from PPI use result in increased levels of amyloid-beta in the brain. Amyloid-beta deposits are proteins that clump together, and when this happens, it can lead to Alzheimer's disease. Even short-term use of PPIs can damage your cognitive abilities, possibly due to these drugs blocking vitamin B12 absorption.

In one study of 60 people, different PPIs significantly reduced visual memory (information you remember about what you've seen) to varying degrees. PPIs also reduced attention span and executive function—a measurement of the ability to plan and organize, remember details, switch focus, and manage time.

Drugs That Lead to Increased Nutrient Loss

Common Painkillers

Acetaminophen (Tylenol), which is in most people's medicine cabinets, lowers levels of glutathione, the most abundant antioxidant inside the cells of the body. Glutathione deficiency spells trouble for the body. It weakens immune response[17] and leads to cell damage that can't be reversed. This damage occurs when a cell is unable to maintain intracellular glutathione levels.[18] Glutathione levels naturally decrease with age. Throwing anything else into the mix (such as acetaminophen) to further deplete glutathione can worsen the oxidative stress (also known as free radical damage) that occurs in aging.[18]

Aspirin, another common resident in most medicine cabinets, causes urinary excretion of vitamin C (ascorbic acid). This loss of vitamin C may make people more vulnerable to aspirin-related bleeding, especially individuals who already have low levels of this vitamin (such as the elderly).[19] Structural changes in the intestines after taking aspirin lower vitamin C levels in cells lining the intestines and in gastric juice.[20,21] Researchers think this drop in ascorbic acid levels is related to aspirin blocking an enzyme that causes a decline in prostaglandin E2 (PGE2). Low levels of PGE2 are associated with structural changes in the intestines that result in inflammation and free radical damage.

Many studies have shown that vitamin C can protect the GI tract from the damaging effects of aspirin. Supplementing aspirin use with ascorbic acid can protect against gastric lesions, bleeding, and injury to the small intestine.[22,23]

Antibiotics

The aminoglycosides class of antibiotics includes the medications amikacin (Amikin), gentamicin (Garamycin), kanamycin (Kantrex), netilmicin

(Netromycin), streptomycin, and tobramycin (Nebcin). These medications increase the urinary excretion of magnesium, potassium, and calcium,[24] electrolytes that are important to proper kidney function. Deficiency of these nutrients is linked to the kidney damage that can occur when taking this class of antibiotics.

Blood-Pressure Lowering Drugs

Diuretics, calcium antagonists, angiotensin-converting enzyme inhibitors, and beta blockers all increase the excretion of zinc from the body.[25] Additionally, certain beta blockers such as propranolol cause a decline in CoQ10 levels.[26]

Beta blockers are given to protect cardiovascular health, and yet they deplete levels of CoQ10, a critical nutrient for proper cardiovascular function. How ironic is that? Some of CoQ10's important actions include reducing mortality from cardiovascular disease,[27,28] reducing scores on a rating scale of Parkinson's disease severity,[29] protecting against free radical damage, and promoting weight loss in people with non-alcoholic fatty liver disease.[30] CoQ10 accomplishes its health-related benefits by protecting the mitochondria, the energy-generating powerhouses of our cells.

Other common blood pressure medications such as thiazide diuretics are known to siphon away important electrolytes such as potassium and magnesium.[31] In addition, this class of drugs may cause a loss of thiamine (vitamin B1).

Drugs That Alter Effects of Nutrients

Antibiotics

Some cephalosporin antibiotics as well as the antibiotic trimethoprim/sulfamethoxazole can stop your body from producing a vitamin K-dependent clotting factor and can cause vitamin K deficiency.[32] Because vitamin K plays an important role in clotting, deficiency of this nutrient can lead to gastrointestinal bleeding. Low vitamin K levels also indicate greater risk of bone fractures and osteoporosis.[33]

Calcium buildup on the arteries leads to atherosclerosis, known as "hardening of the arteries." The extent of vascular calcification predicts morbidity and mortality from cardiovascular disease.[34,35] In other words, it increases risk of death due to heart problems. Calcium deposits on the arteries can be reduced with vitamin K supplementation.

Antiretrovirals

Antiretroviral drugs are used to treat patients with human immunodeficiency virus (HIV). The antiretroviral drug zidovudine (Retrovir), which is also used to treat cancer, weakens the ability of the mitochondria to transport the amino acid L-carnitine into muscle cells, producing low muscle carnitine levels and making the patient more susceptible to muscle weakness.[36] Zidovudine worsens the low carnitine levels already seen in many HIV patients before they begin taking the drug. Supplementation with acetyl-L-carnitine may reduce the free radical damage associated with antiretroviral drugs.[37]

Vitamin D is also negatively affected by antiretroviral drug therapy. Scientists have found that antiretroviral drugs and glucocorticoids (a class of steroid hormones) can damage bone by interfering with the ways bone-building cells known as osteoblasts use vitamin D.[38]

Statin Drugs

Statin drugs, prescribed to lower cholesterol levels, alter the metabolism of CoQ10. Statins interfere with the production of mevalonic acid, a precursor of CoQ10. This is true for all statins, including atorvastatin (Lipitor), fluvastatin (Lescol), lovastatin (Mevacor), pravastatin (Pravachol), rosuvastatin (Crestor), and simvastatin (Zocor).

The drop in CoQ10 levels that occurs with statin use is linked to the muscle-related symptoms that afflict some statin users, including a type of muscle pain known as myopathy. In some studies, CoQ10 supplementation eased this muscle pain. In one study, CoQ10 supplementation reduced statin-related muscle pain in 75% of patients.[39]

Drugs That Are More Toxic in Genetically Susceptible Individuals

Some drugs are more harmful to people who have a genetic defect that causes one or more nutrients to be poorly absorbed by the body. They just don't absorb some nutrients as well as people who do not have this genetic mutation.

Methotrexate, a drug used to treat rheumatoid arthritis, psoriasis, and other autoimmune diseases binds to the enzyme dihydrofolate reductase, preventing the conversion of folate to its active form. A large portion of the world's population have mutations that make their bodies unable to convert folate to its more bioavailable form. These people do not respond well to methotrexate treatment.[40]

Drug Side Effects Worsen with Nutrient Deficiency

Vitamin D deficiency may increase the risk of myopathy in people with high cholesterol who are treated with a low-dose combination of the statin drug atorvastatin and the non-statin cholesterol drug ezetimibe (Zetia). Normally, statin drugs only cause myopathy at higher doses, and ezetimibe rarely causes muscle problems. Vitamin D deficiency may trigger the development of muscular symptoms in people taking these two drugs at the same time, even at a low dose.[41]

Vitamin D or magnesium deficiency can also exacerbate one side effect of zoledronate, a drug used to treat the high calcium levels that happen in malignancy, multiple myeloma, and bone metastases from solid tumors. Although zoledronate normally slows the release of calcium from bones, one possible side effect is lower calcium levels, especially in people with deficiencies in vitamin D or magnesium.[42]

Dietary Supplements Interfering with Drugs

On their own, quality dietary supplements are safe. Compared to pharmaceutical drugs, they have an enviable safety record. But combining certain supplements with specific drugs can interfere with a drug's function. Always check with your 21st Century Pharmacist or healthcare provider to find out if there are any supplements that interact with medicines you may take.

Here are some of the interactions that can occur:

- Magnesium can interfere with the absorption of some antibiotics, such as the quinolone class of drugs.[43]

- Some antibiotics can increase sun sensitivity (known as photo-sensitivity) when taken in conjunction with St. John's wort.[44] St. John's wort can also make birth control pills less effective.[45]

- Some supplements, including Ginkgo biloba, goldenseal, vitamin E, and garlic, act as blood thinners and can potentially increase bleeding when taken in conjunction with anticoagulant drugs.

It's important to develop a good relationship with your 21st Century Pharmacist who is familiar with the potential for these interactions.

Drug-Drug Interactions

We can't emphasize enough the importance of filling all prescriptions at one pharmacy. This way, the pharmacist can monitor all the drugs you may be taking and how they interact with each other. There are thousands of these types of interactions, and I can't cover all of them in this book, but here are some examples:

- Non-steroidal anti-inflammatory drugs (NSAIDs) including OTC drugs like aspirin and ibuprofen boost levels of the medication lithium and prevent lithium clearance from the kidneys.[46] This can increase lithium toxicity, which can result in many problems such as seizures, hallucinations, muscle stiffness, and even death.

- Combining the antibiotic co-trimoxazole with blood pressure-lowering ACE inhibitor drugs such as lisinopril or angiotensin receptor-blocking drugs such as valsartan can cause potassium levels to skyrocket (hyperkalemia), increasing the risk of heart rhythm abnormalities that can lead to death. In one study, people who took this antibiotic with one of these blood-pressure lowering drugs were nearly 7x more likely to end up in the hospital for problems associated with elevated potassium compared to people who were prescribed different antibiotics.[47]

Many of the drug-drug interactions that occur can be life-threatening. That's why having a good 21st Century Pharmacist can literally save your life.

The bottom line is that pharmaceutical drugs may be the accepted way to treat disease, but they are not always safe. Tested and certified dietary supplements have an extremely safe track record. In the next chapter, I'll talk about why the right kinds of nutritional supplements are necessary to feel healthy and full of energy.

Chapter 3 OptiNotes

- Prescriptions and OTC medications routinely come with a fairly long list of side effects.
- Body chemistry changes caused by medications can work for both good and bad.
- 1 in 5 drugs will cause a serious reaction **after** FDA approval.
- Millions of people are hospitalized each year due to properly prescribed prescription medications. Over 100,000 of these people die yearly, making properly prescribed prescription drugs one of the leading causes of death in America.
- Drugs can cause severe nutrient depletions, one of their most serious side effects.
- Drugs can lower nutrient absorption, lead to nutrient loss, or alter the effects of nutrients in the body.
- Some drugs are more toxic in genetically susceptible individuals.
- Nutrient depletion can worsen the side effects of some drugs.
- It is important to fill all prescriptions at one pharmacy where a pharmacist can monitor all drugs and their interactions.

References

1. Harvard University. http://ethics.harvard.edu/blog/new-prescription-drugs-major-health-risk-few-offsetting-advantages Accessed November 7, 2016.

2. O'Shaughnessy K. Principles of clinical pharmacology and drug therapy. Oxford Textbook of Medicine (5 ed.) September 2016. 10.1093/med/9780199204854.003.10

3. Natural Medicine Comprehensive Database. http://naturaldatabase.therapeuticresearch.com/ce/ceCourse.aspx?pc=08-40&cec=0 &pm=5&AspxAutoDetectCookieSupport=1 Accessed November 7, 2016.

4. Lambie DG, Johnson RH. Drugs. 1985 Aug;30(2):145-55.

5. Roy RP, et al. Indian J Endocrinol Metab. 2016 Sep-Oct;20(5):631-7.

6. Tomkin GH, et al. Br Med J. 1971 Jun 19;2(5763):685-7.

7. Bauman WA, et al. Diabetes Care. 2000 Sep;23(9):1227-31.

8. Singh C, et al. Noise Health. 2016 Mar-Apr;18(81):93-7.

9. Gupta L, et al. Magn Reson Imaging. 2016 Feb;34(2):191-6.

10. Kwok T, et al. J Nutr Health Aging. 2012;16(6):569-73.

11. Kurt R, et al. Arch Med Res. 2010 Jul;41(5):369-72.

12. Ago R, et al. Hemodial Int. 2016 Oct;20(4):580-8.

13. Rozgony NR, et al. J Nutr Elder. 2010 Jan;29(1):87-99.

14. Liamis G, et al. J Bone Miner Metab. 2009;27(6):635-42.

15. Hansen BA, Bruserud Ø. Oxf Med Case Reports. 2016 Jul 27;2016(7):147-9.

16. Akter S, et al. Alzheimers Res Ther. 2015 Dec 27;7:79.

17. Tan KS, et al. J Clin Invest. 2012 Jun;122(6):2289-300.

18. Sekhar RV, et al. Am J Clin Nutr. 2011 Sep;94(3):847-53.

19. Coffey G, Wilson CW. Br Med J. 1975 Jan 25;1(5951):208.

20. Buffinton GD, Doe WF. Free Radical Res. 1995;22:131-43.

21. Pohle T, et al. Aliment Pharmacol Ther. 2001;15:677-87.

22. Konturek PC, et al. J Physiol Pharmacol. 2006 Nov;57 Suppl 5:125-36.

23. Pohle T, et al. Aliment Pharmacol Ther. 2001 May;15(5):677-87.

24. Heydari B, et al. Iran J Pharm Res. 2016 Spring;15(2):627-34.

25. Suliburska J, et al. Eur Rev Med Pharmacol Sci. 2014;18(1):58-65.

26. Sarter B. J Cardiovasc Nurs. 2002 Jul;16(4):9-20.

27. Alehagen U, et al. PLoS One. 2015 Dec 1;10(12):e0141641.

28. Mortensen SA, et al. JACC Heart Fail. 2014 Dec;2(6):641-9.

29. Yoritaka A, et al. Parkinsonism Relat Disord. 2015 Aug;21(8):911-6.

30. Farhangi MA, et al. Arch Med Res. 2014 Oct;45(7):589-95.

31. Ruml LA, et al. Am J Ther. 1999 Jan;6(1):45-50.

32. Fotouhie A, et al. BMJ Case Rep. Published Online 6 June 2016; doi:10.1136/bcr-2016-214437.

33. Inaba N, et al. J Nutr Sci Vitaminol (Tokyo). 2015;61(6):471-80.

34. Vossen LM, et al. Nutrients. 2015 Oct 28;7(11):8905-15.

35. Westenfeld R, et al. Am J Kidney Dis. 2012 Feb;59(2):186-95.

36. Scruggs ER, Dirks Naylor AJ. Pharmacology. 2008;82(2):83-8.

37. Ferraresi R, et al. FEBS Lett. 2006 Dec 11;580(28-29):6612-6.

38. Wegler C, et al. Basic Clin Pharmacol Toxicol. 2016 Nov;119(5):436-42.

39. Skarlovnik A, et al. Med Sci Monit. 2014 Nov 6;20:2183-8.

40. Lima A, et al. Biomed Res Int. 2014;2014:368681.

41. Brahmachari B, Chatterjee S. Indian J Pharmacol. 2015 Sep-Oct;47(5):563-4.

42. Epperla N, Pathak R. WMJ. 2015 Aug;114(4):163-6.

43. Imaoka A, et al. Drug Metab Pharmacokinet. 2014;29(5):414-8.

44. Wilhelm KP, et al. Phytomedicine. 2001 Jul;8(4):306-9.

45. Berry-Bibee EN, et al. Contraception. 2016 Jul 18. [Epub ahead of print.]

46. Hassan S, et al. Case Rep Nephrol. 2013;2013:839796.

47. Antoniou T, et al. Arch Intern Med. 2010 Jun 28;170(12):1045-9.

CHAPTER 4

Are Dietary Supplements Harming or Helping Your Health?

L et's talk about supplements. Do you really need them? And how do you know that you're really getting what you pay for? Do you know if you're getting the best quality possible?

A lot of medical journal research supports the use of dietary supplements. I'll show you some of that research in this chapter. The science proves that quality supplements can make you healthier, give you more energy, and fend off disease. Doctors often ignore this research. Why? Mainly because, as I mentioned earlier, medical school taught them that pharmaceutical drugs are the only answer.

It's a catch-22 situation. Doctors prescribe drugs to treat an illness. These drugs decrease the nutrient levels needed to stay healthy. As these levels nosedive, health suffers. Does this make sense to you?

It never made sense to me.

I remember it like it was yesterday; a lovely couple named Ida and James began visiting Prescriptions Plus. They were in the pharmacy **a lot.** Both were diabetics and suffered from many of the complications often associated with this disease. Ida was taking 15 different prescription drugs, and James was on 12. They had no energy and a low quality of life. I knew this could be improved with some simple changes. Using the right supplements could at least offset some of the nutritional deficiencies from their poor diet and drug regimens.

Unfortunately, the couple's doctor told them supplements wouldn't help. They believed it was a waste of money and continued to suffer from lack of energy, aches, pains, and other issues that made day-to-day life difficult.

Yes, You Need Supplements

According to the CDC, 76% of people in the U.S. do not eat the recommended 1.5 to 2 cups of fruit daily, and 87% do not eat the recommended 2 to 3 cups of vegetables daily.[1] Most of us are starving ourselves of important nutrients!

Even the fruits and vegetables we do consume are low in the nutrients needed by the body. Today's food isn't nearly as nutritious as it was when our grandparents were growing up. Modern farming practices deplete nutrients from the soil in which fruits and vegetables are grown.

Today's crops are bred to produce a greater yield, be resistant to pests, and adapt to poor climate conditions. These crops grow bigger and faster, but the ability to make nutrients or pull them from the soil cannot keep up with the accelerated growth.

Researchers from the University of Texas found evidence of this when they studied the nutrient contents of 43 crops (mostly vegetables) between 1950 and 1999.[2] They found a significant drop in levels of protein, calcium, phosphorus, iron, riboflavin, and vitamin C in produce from 1999 when compared to the crops from 1950, with riboflavin levels dropping the most dramatically.

The researchers believe levels of other nutrients such as magnesium, zinc, and vitamins B6 and E also declined in the crops, but the United States Department of Agriculture (USDA) did not gather data on these nutrients in 1950.

Other studies have yielded similar conclusions. One study claims that between 1975 and 1997, average calcium levels in 12 fresh vegetables fell by 27%. Iron levels fell by 37%, vitamin A levels by 21%, and vitamin C levels by 30%.[3] You'd need to eat **eight** oranges to get the same amount of vitamin A as your grandparents got with just one! Eight to one! That's a lot of oranges in one day.

Can you understand why you need a high-quality multivitamin to make up for the nutrients missing from your diet? It's no wonder that the Physicians' Health Study II found that multivitamin supplementation was linked to a 39% drop in the risk of heart attack.[4] Another study of healthy men found that taking a multivitamin for 20 or more years was linked to having a lesser risk of cardiovascular problems.[5]

The benefits of multivitamins don't stop there. Scientists reported that multivitamins reduce the risk of developing colorectal cancer.[6] Another study found that taking a daily multivitamin can increase energy levels and improve mood and sleep.[7] Multivitamins have also been shown to improve memory in older men at risk of cognitive decline.[8]

What Research Says About Some Dietary Supplement Ingredients	
Benfotiamine	Reduces dependence on alcohol in alcoholics,[9] protects against toxic compounds known as advanced glycation end-products (AGEs),[10] and stops damage to blood vessels in peripheral neuropathy, a painful nerve condition.[11]
Selenium	Stops precancerous and abnormal growth of cervical cells,[12] benefits people with autoimmune thyroiditis,[13] improves the body's ability to use insulin, lowers triglycerides and an especially harmful form of "bad" cholesterol known as very low density lipoprotein cholesterol in women with polycystic ovary syndrome.[14] Important for prostate health.[15]
Chromium	Improves the body's ability to use glucose (blood sugar) in type 2 diabetics with poorly controlled disease.[16] Causes significant drop in levels of HbA1c, a marker for healthy blood sugar control in the same patients.
Vitamin D3	Beneficial in people with Hashimoto's thyroiditis,[17] polycystic ovary syndrome,[18] coronary artery disease,[19] and multiple sclerosis.[20] Reduces number of falls in elderly women.[21]

Thiamin	Reduces mental and physical symptoms of pre-menstrual syndrome (PMS).[22] Improves the body's ability to use glucose and insulin.[23] Improves memory in people detoxifying from alcohol.[24]
Biotin	Beneficial in multiple sclerosis patients.[25] Reduces muscle cramps in people with poor kidney function on hemodialysis.[26] Lowers levels of "bad" cholesterol (low-density lipoprotein cholesterol) and improves body use of glucose when combined with chromium.[27]
Magnesium	Improves sleep.[28] Increases energy, improves mood, and reduces pain in patients with chronic fatigue.[29] Supports healthy blood pressure levels.[30]
Coenzyme Q10 (CoQ10)	Reduces inflammation in people with high blood pressure.[31] When combined with selenium, lowers risk of death from cardiovascular disease.[32] Reduces free radical damage and inflammation in rheumatoid arthritis patients.[33] Decreases risk of developing abnormal heart rhythm (atrial fibrillation) in heart failure patients when used with drugs commonly prescribed to treat this condition.[34] Beneficial for athletes participating in strenuous exercise.[35]

Meet Your Friendly Flora

Beneficial bacteria live throughout your body and in your intestines. The population of these bacteria, along with bad bacteria and other tiny organisms, is known as microbiota. The good bacteria are involved in supporting your health in a surprising number of ways. But these bacteria are constantly under attack, killed by antibiotics in the pills we take to fight infections and in the meat we eat (unless it's organic). This creates an imbalance where the bad bacteria outnumber the good bacteria, leading to disease.

Antibiotics aren't the only killer of good bacteria. Stress can weaken these friendly flora, too.[36] A high-sugar diet can also wreak havoc on your good bacteria.[37] So can exposure to the toxin bisphenol-A (BPA).[37] You're exposed to a lot of BPA everywhere, from plastic containers to metal cans and even cash register receipts. Touching a receipt and then eating exposes you to this toxin.

Microbiota also change with age. Age-related intestinal and memory problems and immune system damage are all linked to imbalance between good and bad bacteria.[38] Imbalance in the microbiota is linked to many additional health problems including obesity, multiple sclerosis, memory problems, and heart disease.[39-42]

That's why it's so important to take a probiotic supplement. My probiotic formula contains good bacteria such as *Lactobacillus* and *Bifidobacterium*. Thousands of studies in animals and humans show that probiotics are necessary for health. I don't have room to discuss all the results from those studies, but here are some highlights:

- A meta-analysis of studies on the impact of probiotics on mental health found that people who took probiotics were less anxious, stressed, and depressed. Can you imagine reducing all of these factors with just one supplement?

- A clinical trial of 110 people found that taking the probiotic *Lactobacillus plantarum* increased skin hydration. What's more, wrinkles in people taking the probiotic were less deep, and their skin was glossier than people who weren't taking the probiotics. Skin elasticity (the ability of the skin to stretch and return to normal, which declines with age) also improved in the probiotic group.[44]

- Researchers gave 49 patients with irritable bowel syndrome (IBS) either a probiotic containing *Bifidobacterium longum*,

Bifidobacterium bifidum, Bifidobacterium lactis, Lactobacillus acidophilus, Lactobacillus rhamnosus, and *Streptococcus thermophilus* or a placebo twice daily for four weeks. IBS symptoms went away in more patients in the probiotic group than the placebo group. Abdominal pain/discomfort and bloating improved in people taking the probiotic but not the placebo.[45]

- *L. plantarum* reduced probing depth in a study of 39 patients with gum disease.[46] Gum disease causes tissue detachment, creating a pocket. Probing depth refers to the deepness of this pocket.

- In people with cirrhosis of the liver, the probiotic *Lactobacillus GG* reduced bacterial toxins in the blood.[47]

- College students taking the probiotic *Lactobacillus casei* experienced fewer abdominal and common cold symptoms than peers taking a placebo during exam stress. Students taking the probiotic also had higher levels of the feel-good hormone serotonin.[48]

Do Probiotics Really Need to Be Refrigerated?

Many people have heard that probiotics should be refrigerated because they are live and refuse to trust probiotics that are sold at room temperature. Products that are sold as refrigerated are really just marketing and posturing to be regarded as premium. In reality, if a probiotic can't live at room temperature (about 73.4°F), then it cannot live to take effect in your body—the average body temperature is 98.6°F!

The Foundational Four

As part of my ongoing mission to help people obtain optimal health, I enlisted the help of a leading doctor and a professional formulator to create four proprietary supplements that I believe are absolutely fundamental to basic health.

1. Multivitamin. Studies have shown that taking a multivitamin can reduce your risk of heart disease and colorectal cancer, improve

your mood and energy, and make up for diets that don't include enough fruits and vegetables.

2. Magnesium. This mineral has over 300 positive functions in the body![76] Included in those are its ability to improve sleep, reduce migraines and nighttime leg cramps, reduce blood pressure, and support cardiovascular health.

3. Probiotic. Taking a high-quality probiotic supplement can improve mood, reduce IBS symptoms, improve the health of your gums, hydrate your skin, support brain health, and much, much more.

4. Digestive Enzymes. These enzymes reduce the need for heartburn and acid reflux medications by breaking down food so that your body can more easily utilize the fats, proteins, and carbohydrates you intake properly. Digestive enzymes can help with weight loss as well.

The truth is, when someone tells you that taking dietary supplements won't do you any good, research simply does not support what they are saying. The important thing is that you realize not all supplements are created equal. It is essential to choose high-quality supplements.

Always remember: the most expensive supplement is the one that does not work—or harms you!

Inferior quality supplements can **harm** your health instead of helping it. Some contain toxic ingredients. Others, when tested, do not even contain their listed active ingredients!

What should you look for when choosing a dietary supplement? And how can you know what you're being told is the truth?

Is Your Multivitamin Damaging Your Health?

If you currently take many of the bestselling multivitamins, the answer to that question is "yes." One of the perennial bestsellers is made by the same pharmaceutical company that brings us one of the most popular statin drugs. Representatives pass out samples of this multi at doctors' offices, so guess which multivitamin doctors often recommend? That's right: the very same one.

But is this product really the best multivitamin on the market? Let's take a look at the ingredients.

First, the dosages of the nutrients in this particular bestseller are particularly low, and many of the nutrient forms are not absorbed maximally by the body. I'll talk more about the nutrients that your body absorbs best later in this chapter.

The worst part about this formula is that it contains toxic fillers, binders, and texturizers, including talc. Sadly, this is not unique amongst popular multivitamin products. What's wrong with talc? It comes with a possible increased risk of cancer.[49] Inhaling talc can also cause a type of cancer called mesothelioma, which has been linked to asbestos exposure. Understandable, considering talc sometimes contains asbestos.[50]

The research showing talc is linked to cancer involved subjects who breathed it in. But clearly, it's not a health-promoting substance regardless of delivery method. It isn't something that anyone with a discerning mind who wants to feel better should ingest.

Two different food colorings are also in this product. Yellow 6 Lake, also called tartrazine or FD&C Yellow #6, is a combination of benzenesulfonic acid, hydrochloric acid, and sodium nitrite. Norway and Finland have banned Yellow 6 Lake—and with good reason. It's one of a number of food additives suspected of causing hyperactivity in young children according to some studies.[51]

One study found that when children eat Yellow 6 Lake, they're more irritable and restless and suffer from more sleep problems when compared to eating a placebo.[52] In some people, Yellow 6 Lake can cause skin rashes, a severe swelling beneath the skin known as angioedema, stomach upset, diarrhea, vomiting, headaches, migraines, problems concentrating, and joint pain.[53]

The food coloring Red 40 Lake is also found in this bestselling formula. Red 40 Lake contains the chemical compounds benzidine and

4-aminobiphenyl. Being exposed to benzidine over long periods increases your risk of developing bladder cancer as well as cancer of the small intestine and cancer in soft tissue including the heart.[54,55]

4-aminobiphenyl is also a known carcinogen. It causes liver cancer in rodents.[56] In humans, it is known, like benzidine, to cause bladder cancer.[57] Is this really something you want in your multivitamin?

Here's a breakdown of some of the other disturbing ingredients in this formula:

- Hydrogenated palm oil. Palm oil in its natural state isn't so bad for you. But once it's been hydrogenated, it becomes toxic. Hydrogenated oils are heated from 500 to 1,000 degrees. Then a metal such as nickel, platinum, or aluminum is injected into the heated oil. The molecular structure of the oil changes and increases in density, becoming solid oil. At this point, its molecular structure more closely resembles plastic than oil. Consumption of this substance thickens blood and increases the risk of heart problems.

Studies in rodents have found that eating hydrogenated oil shortens the survival of rats with high blood pressure that are prone to having strokes. Hydrogenated oil also damages kidney function. Palm oil specifically is linked to the development of colon cancer.[58]

- Sodium benzoate. This synthetic preservative is known to damage DNA.[59,60] Anything that damages your DNA is not something you want to put in your body. Excessive DNA damage will speed up aging and cause many other health problems.
- Sodium aluminosilicate. This food additive is a source of aluminum. Aluminum intake increases the risk of developing dementia.[61] Long-term exposure to aluminum through drinking water leads to aluminum buildup in the brain, which causes cognitive and memory problems. I think it's safe to assume that this substance is no better when ingested via this bestselling multivitamin than via drinking water.

Numerous studies have shown that aluminum is toxic to the brain. In one study where mice were exposed to aluminum, the rodents displayed memory problems and the inability to socialize well with other mice.[62] In another study, researchers fed rats the same amount of aluminum, leading to memory problems.[63]

Alzheimer's patients who are not given a treatment to lower aluminum levels get worse twice as fast as those who are given an aluminum-lowering treatment.[64]

This toxic cocktail of ingredients is not what you want to find in your multivitamin, and this particular product actually contains more of these unhealthy ingredients than it does beneficial vitamins and minerals!

Absorbing Multivitamins

Most multivitamins contain forms of nutrients that your body simply can't absorb very well. Folic acid shows up on the label of many multivitamin formulas. The problem is that many people—and you could be one of them—have a genetic mutation that prevents them from converting folic acid into its more absorbable form. This means folic acid as an ingredient does these people absolutely no good. Up to 40% of the American population has been estimated to be affected.

If you're one of the people who can't absorb folic acid, not only are you throwing money down the drain by buying a multivitamin with folic acid, you're putting your health at risk. That's because folate (the active form of folic acid) is necessary for the health of your heart, your brain, and many other areas of your body. That's why your multivitamin should contain 5-methyltetrahydrofolate. Unlike folic acid, which needs to be changed into the active form of folate, 5-methyltetrahydrofolate is already the active form of this vitamin. This means your body absorbs it much better.[65]

A good multivitamin should also contain:

- Pyridoxal 5'-phosphate (P5P). P5P is a form of vitamin B6 that is easier for your body to absorb. P5P is the coenzyme form of B6.

A coenzyme is a compound that an enzyme requires to work properly. P5P is a coenzyme for more than 150 enzymes in the human body. Low levels of P5P are linked to heart disease, some cancers, and inflammation.[66]

- Natural vitamin E. Always make sure your multivitamin contains natural vitamin E, listed as d-alpha tocopherol, d-alpha tocopherol acetate, or d-alpha tocopherol succinate. Avoid forms of vitamin E labeled with the "dl" prefix since these are synthetic. Researchers found that the human body excretes synthetic vitamin E three times faster than natural vitamin E.[67] Another study showed natural vitamin E increased twice as much as synthetic vitamin E in the blood and tissue of people taking vitamin E supplements.[68]

- Magnesium aspartate, taurinate, malate, succinate, and citrate. Supplementing with these organic forms of magnesium greatly improves the absorption of the mineral compared with inorganic forms such as magnesium oxide, sulfate, chloride, and carbonate.[69] In a 60-day trial on 46 healthy individuals, magnesium citrate resulted in greater absorption than the inorganic magnesium oxide and resulted in the highest blood and saliva magnesium levels.[70] In fact, supplementing with magnesium oxide was no better than a placebo at raising magnesium levels.

- Methylcobalamin, the active form of vitamin B12. Some dietary supplements use another form of B12 known as cyanocobalamin. The problem with cyanocobalamin is the body's inability to optimally use it. The body must work extra hard to convert cyanocobalamin into the active form of vitamin B12: methylcobalamin. Even worse, cyanocobalamin can harm people whose kidneys aren't working properly.[71,72] This is because the cyanide in cyanocobalamin builds up in the bodies of these people.

Methylcobalamin is the best form of vitamin B12. It's also the only form of vitamin B12 that can cross what's known as **the blood-brain**

barrier, which stops toxins from entering the brain. An unfortunate side effect is the blood-brain barrier's ability to also stop some beneficial substances from crossing the barrier, but methylcobalamin can make it through. This may explain why methylcobalamin has helped people with ALS and multiple sclerosis.[73,74]

Methylcobalamin can also help lower levels of homocysteine, an amino acid linked to heart disease and stroke as well as many other diseases. This form of vitamin B12 converts the damaging homocysteine to harmless methionine.[75]

Choosing the Best Supplements

It is important to make sure your dietary supplements are safe and work properly. Always look for supplements produced in a Current Good Manufacturing Practices (cGMP) registered facility. This means the manufacturer meets FDA-enforced guidelines comparable to prescription drug regulations. cGMP guidelines ensure that a supplement's identity, potency, composition, quality, and purity match what appears on its label.

Also check whether your supplements are manufactured in an NSF International GMP registered facility. NSF International serves as an independent watchdog that makes sure manufacturers are meeting cGMP requirements at all times.

Both of these stipulations are **optional** for manufacturers and brands, so be sure that you deal with a transparent supplement distributor who puts your health and wellness above the bottom line.

Delivery Method

Finally, I'll answer the age-old debate: which is better, tablets or capsules? In many cases, tablets pass through the digestive tract without breaking down and releasing the nutrients contained within. Tablets also contain many excipients (fillers). That's why we prefer capsules, and my supplement line comes in capsule form.

Chapter 4 OptiNotes

- Doctors are skeptical about supplements because they have not received proper training. The idea that "supplements are worthless" is not backed by research.

- Prescription drugs deplete nutrients that can be replaced by supplements.

- According to the CDC, people don't get enough dietary nutrients, and even healthy food today is less healthy than it used to be.

- Studies have shown quality multivitamins decrease the risk of cardiovascular issues and have many other benefits.

- The beneficial bacteria in your body are killed by antibiotics—not just via medication but also through food. Imbalance between good and bad bacteria leads to many health problems, which is why probiotics are so essential.

- There are Four Foundational Supplements: multivitamin, magnesium, probiotic, and digestive enzymes.

- Get quality supplements. Some are filled with toxins, binders, and fillers—doing more harm than good. Demand quality and honesty by purchasing supplements produced in a cGMP facility that is NSF International registered.

References

1. Centers for Disease Control and Prevention. http://www.cdc.gov/mmwr/preview/mmwrhtml/mm6426a1.htm Accessed on December 28, 2016.

2. Davis DR, et al. J Am Coll Nutr. 2004 Dec;23(6):669-82.

3. Scientific American. https://www.scientificamerican.com/article/soil-depletion-and-nutrition-loss/ Accessed on December 28, 2016.

4. Sesso HD, et al. JAMA. 2012;308:1751-60.

5. Rautiainen S, et al. J Nutr. 2016;146:1235-40.

6. Heine-Bröring RC, et al. Int J Cancer. 2015;136:2388-401.

7. Sarris J, et al. Nutr J. 2012 Dec 14;11:110.

8. Harris E, et al. Hum Psychopharmacol. 2012 Jul;27(4):370-7.

9. Manzardo AM, et al. Drug Alcohol Depend. 2013 Dec 1;133(2):562-70.

10. Nenna A, et al. Res Cardiovasc Med. 2015 May 23;4(2):e26949.

11. Javed S, et al. Diabetes Obes Metab. 2015 Dec;17(12):1115-25.

12. Karamali M, et al. Br J Nutr. 2015 Dec 28;114(12):2039-45.

13. de Farias CR, et al. J Endocrinol Invest. 2015 Oct;38(10):1065-74.

14. Jamilian M, et al. Clin Endocrinol (Oxf). 2015 Jun;82(6):885-91.

15. Clark LC, et al. Br J Urol. 1998 May;81(5):730-4.

16. Paiva AN, et al. J Trace Elem Med Biol. 2015 Oct;32:66-72.

17. Mazokopakis EE, et al. Hell J Nucl Med. 2015 Sep-Dec;18(3):222-7.

18. Irani M, et al. J Clin Endocrinol Metab. 2015 Nov;100(11):4307-14.

19. Wu Z, et al. Scand Cardiovasc J. 2016;50(1):9-16.

20. Ashtari F, et al. Neuroimmunomodulation. 2015;22(6):400-4.

21. Cangussu LM, et al. Menopause. 2016 Mar;23(3):267-74.

22. Abdollahifard S, et al. Glob J Health Sci. 2014 Jul 29;6(6):144-53.

23. Alaei Shahmiri F, et al. Eur J Nutr. 2013 Oct;52(7):1821-4.

24. Ambrose ML, et al. Alcohol Clin Exp Res. 2001 Jan;25(1):112-6.

25. Sedel F, et al. Mult Scler Relat Disord. 2015 Mar;4(2):159-69.

26. Oguma S, et al. Tohoku J Exp Med. 2012;227(3):217-23.

27. Albarracin C, et al. Cardiometab Syndr. 2007 Spring;2(2):91-7.

28. Held K, et al. Pharmacopsychiatry. 2002 Jul;35(4):135-43.

29. Cox IM, et al. Lancet. 1991 Mar 30;337(8744):757-60.

30. Hatzistavri LS, et al. Am J Hypertens. 2009 Oct;22(10):1070-5.

31. Bagheri Nesami N, et al. Int J Vitam Nutr Res. 2015;85(3-4):156-64.

32. Alehagen U, et al. PLoS One. 2015 Dec 1;10(12):e0141641.

33. Abdollahzad H, et al. Arch Med Res. 2015 Oct;46(7):527-33.

34. Zhao Q, et al. J Investig Med. 2015 Jun;63(5):735-9.

35. Shimizu K, et al. Appl Physiol Nutr Metab. 2015 Jun;40(6):575-81.

36. Gur TL, Bailey MT.Adv Exp Med Biol. 2016;874:289-300.

37. Lai KP, et al. Environ Pollut. 2016 Nov;218:923-930.

38. Salazar N, et al. Gut Microbes. 2016 Nov 3:1-16. [Epub ahead of print.]

39. Zhang C, et al. EBioMedicine. 2015 Jul 10;2(8):968-84.

40. Miyake S, et al. PLoS One. 2015 Sep 14;10(9):e0137429.

41. Gareau MG. Int Rev Neurobiol. 2016;131:227-246.

42. Yamashita T. J Atheroscler Thromb. 2016 Dec 7. [Epub ahead of print.]

43. McKean J, et al. J Altern Complement Med. 2016 Nov 14. [Epub ahead of print.]

44. Lee DE, et al. J Microbiol Biotechnol. 2015 Dec 28;25(12):2160-8.

45. Yoon JS, et al. J Gastroenterol Hepatol. 2014 Jan;29(1):52-9.

46. Iwasaki K, et al. Oral Health Prev Dent. 2016;14(3):207-14.

47. Bajaj JS, et al. Aliment Pharmacol Ther. 2014 May;39(10):1113-25.

48. Kato-Kataoka A, et al. Benef Microbes. 2016;7(2):153-6.

49. Wentzensen N, Wacholder S. J Natl Cancer Inst. 2014 Sep 10;106(9). pii: dju260.

50. Gordon RE, et al. Int J Occup Environ Health.2014 Oct;20(4):318-32.

51. Bateman B, et al. Arch Dis Child. 2004 Jun;89(6):506-11.

52. Rowe KS, Rowe KJ. J Pediatr. 1994 Nov;125(5 Pt 1):691-8.

53. Novembre E, et al. Pediatr Med Chir. 1992 Jan-Feb;14(1):39-42.

54. Sun X, et al. Exp Toxicol Pathol. 2016 Apr;68(4):215-22.

55. Brown SC, et al. Am J Ind Med. 2011 Apr;54(4):300-6.

56. Wang S, et al. Toxicol Sci. 2015 Apr;144(2):393-405.

57. Tao L, et al. Cancer Epidemiol Biomarkers Prev. 2013 May;22(5): 937-45.

58. Okuyama H, et al. Pharmacology. 2016;98(3-4):134-70.

59. Pongsavee M. Biomed Res Int. 2015;2015:103512.

60. Zengin N, et al. Food Chem Toxicol. 2011 Apr;49(4):763-9.

61. Cao L, et al. Mol Neurobiol. 2016 Nov;53(9):6144-54.

62. Farhat SM, et al. Biol Trace Elem Res. 2016 Oct 6. [Epub ahead of print.]

63. Martinez CS, et al. Neurotox Res. 2016 Jul 29. [Epub ahead of print.]

64. McLachlan DR, et al. Ther Drug Monit. 1993 Dec;15(6):602-7.

65. Pietrzik K, et al. Clin Pharmacokinet. 2010 Aug;49(8):535-48.

66. Ueland PM, et al. Mol Aspects Med. 2016 Sep 1. [Epub ahead of print.]

67. Traber MG, et al. FEBS Lett.1998 Oct 16;437(1-2):145-8.

68. Burton GW, et al. Am J Clin Nutr. 1998 Apr;67(4):669-84.

69. Kass LS, Poeira F. J Int Soc Sports Nutr. 2015;12:19.

70. Walker AF, et al. Magnes Res. 2003 Sep;16(3):183-91.

71. Spence JD. Nutr Res. 2016 Feb;36(2):109-16.

72. Spence JD. Clin Chem Lab Med. 2013 Mar 1;51(3):633-7.

73. Izumi Y, Kaji R. Brain Nerve. 2007 Oct;59(10):1141-7.

74. Kira J, et al. Intern Med. 1994 Feb;33(2):82-6.

75. Kozlowski PM, et al. J Biol Inorg Chem. 2012 Apr;17(4):611-9.

76. https://medlineplus.gov/ency/article/002423.htm

CHAPTER 5

Building a Foundation:
What Is OptiYou RX?

What health problem is your biggest challenge? Maybe you're overweight and have trouble shedding those extra pounds. Maybe you're really tired and suffer from fatigue. Perhaps your brain isn't working as well as it used to, and you have memory problems or brain fog. Or maybe you can't sleep, can't relax, are in pain, or don't feel like having sex anymore. Maybe despite your best efforts, your blood sugar is out of control.

Over the last decades I've developed a program that can help. It's called the **OptiYou RX Program.** The program's 12 detailed classes and personalized coaching give participants amazing energy and vigor, shifting their brains from first gear into overdrive and transforming their bodies into fat-burning machines. I wish I could include all of the information the OptiYou RX Program covers in this book, but that would be impossible. The OptiYou RX Program is an intensive and intentional two-day education and experience, a complete package geared to helping participants target their biggest health problems and risk factors. The OptiYou RX Program is backed by science and clinical success in helping thousands eliminate, reverse, and mitigate their health problems. Participants invariably find new energy, vigor, and zest for life and optimal health upon completion of the program. For more information, check out the website *www.optiyourx.com*

By now, you've realized that many of your beliefs and much of what you were taught is completely wrong. You've never had the information you need to change your health and feel your best.

Now you do.

In this chapter, I'll introduce you to the OptiYou RX Program and show you how it can help you achieve a vibrancy and quality of life you could only dream of before.

> *"Billy, thank you. In just 8 weeks on the OptiYou RX Program, I have lost almost 40 pounds, ate more than usual, and most importantly, I am pain-free for the first time in 3 years. I'm off all medications and finally sleeping. You taught me how to eat, how to [grocery] shop, and how to supplement. As I told you when we started, I was a skeptic and went kicking and screaming with my wife. But now if you said eat spiders, I would find a bowl of them. Thank you!"*

> **— Bence**

The OptiYou RX Program is easy to follow, and the science behind it is explained in easy-to-understand terms. The results are mind-blowing. As you'll see from the testimonials and notes from those who've followed it, OptiYou RX works.

If you want these results, you'll have to make some permanent lifestyle changes and follow the OptiYou RX Program forever. But following forever is easy to do once you realize how easy to implement and rewarding it is. After you experience a healthier body and mind, you'll never want to go back.

> *"Billy, just leaving you this note. I went back to the doctor for the first time since starting. My glucose was 290, now it's 69. Hemoglobin was 12.7, and now it's 8.3 Thanks!"*

> **— Willie**

> *"The OptiYou RX course is the BEST thing I have done for my own health in my lifetime! It is not always easy, yet it is absolutely worth it!!! (from one who knows and is sticking to it)!"*

> **— Wanda**

What Is OptiYou RX?

The OptiYou RX Program is not a diet in the usual sense of the word— it's simply healthy eating. It calls for you to eat until full when you are hungry, as long as you stick to the healthy shopping and recipe list my team and I have created. You won't necessarily be eating less, just eating healthier from the choices we provide. We teach you how to properly fuel the body and activate your built-in fat-burning ability. Besides, the OptiYou RX Program is about much more than just what you eat. It's about your entire lifestyle.

Johnny said: *As a participant of the last OptiYou RX Summit, it has been exactly one week since it concluded, and I have lost 8 pounds of fat. To be clear, I am a former professional soccer athlete, and exercise has always been a part of my lifestyle. PAY ATTENTION: I did not exercise at all in this 7 day period. I was actually disappointed in myself for not doing so, yet the fat fell off. Wow! Imagine what would have happened with just 3 days of focused exercise. Oh, did I say that I was never hungry and ate as much of the recommended foods as I wanted. Go to the next free OptiYou RX Wellness Workshop to find out why you should attend the next summit. What do you have to lose by attending? I will tell you what: FAT!!!*

The OptiYou RX Program is supported by my **5 Pillars of Optimal Health.** The science behind these pillars shows you how to boost energy, burn fat, and take on some of your most challenging health problems. I'll go over these Pillars in the next chapter.

In the OptiYou RX Program, we educate you about the best water to drink and how you can get access to it.

> *"I decided to try the water knowing that some counties' drinking water has different levels of toxins in them. I had been having trouble with my kidneys and my bladder and had difficulty swallowing on occasion. My energy levels had been noticeably low, something very unusual for a high-energy person like myself.*
>
> *"At first I was skeptical, but quickly noticed a change in my swallowing. I no longer had trouble with pills getting stuck in my*

throat, something that had been increasingly prevalent in the pre-
vious year. My acid reflux disappeared soon after.

"The next thing I noticed was my energy level. Within 2 to 3
weeks, I felt much better. After being tested, I began adding Billy's
supplements and hormone therapy recommendations. I cancelled
my scheduled bladder surgery because I didn't feel I needed it
any longer. After a recent retest, I can confirm that my bladder
and kidneys are in much better condition than they were a year
ago. My energy level keeps going up, and I'm exercising every day
again. I am much more productive at work and have a better
outlook since I began to feel better.

"I know this water and Billy's recommendations are the reasons
for my improved health and strength. The more I drink, the bet-
ter I feel. You will be amazed at the healing it can bring to your
body."

— Melody

The OptiYou RX Program incorporates a high-fat diet, intermittent fasting, proper supplementation, quality hydration, the most effective exercise, proven success principles, and much more to create a positive environment where optimal health can flourish. There are delicious recipes, shopping lists, and easy ways to incorporate the program even while traveling and on the go.

"In summer 2008, I started a new job despite numerous health
issues like aching joints and excruciating foot pain. My symptoms
worsened as time passed, to the point that it took immense effort
just to get out of bed. After just 15 minutes of inactivity, it was
nearly impossible to get myself going again. I suffered incredible
pain in all my weight-bearing joints and the nerves attached
to them. My doctor prescribed Tramadol, but it didn't help. Noth-
ing did.

"In April 2009, my doctor tested my thyroid and told me that it wasn't a problem because I was in the normal range. I visited two podiatrists who looked at my feet and simply shook their heads. I gave up hope. My skin was dry, my hair was brittle and falling out, I was losing eyelashes, and I had been sick for months on end. I was wrapping my feet in bandages just to be able to move at all. I was so fatigued, I couldn't make it through a normal day of clerical work. After work, I would collapse onto the coach and sleep for around 90 minutes each afternoon. On weekends, I simply lived in bed. My husband took care of the house and helped me out of bed when necessary. By summer 2009, I was 52 years old and had lost my will to live. I begged God to send someone to help me or to take me to heaven. He answered through healing.

"My employer offered after-work courses on various topics. It was one of these classes that saved my life: thyroid and hormone health taught by local pharmacist Billy Wease. As he gave examples of symptoms throughout his presentation, I thought, "That sounds exactly like me!" After the class, I gave him a brief rundown of my problems. He recommended undergoing additional thyroid tests that most practitioners don't offer. In December 2009, I was diagnosed with severe Hashimoto's Disease with antibody levels that staggered even professionals. The normal range was below 60; my count came in at 4,445.9. The technician responsible for the test even ran it multiple times because the number was so unheard of. My vitamin D levels were extremely low, further contributing to my joint problems. I had been taking Synthroid for low thyroid for years, but my body could not convert the medication (T4) into the product our bodies need to function (T3). I discovered I also had celiac disease and was allergic to gluten.

"I finally had a diagnosis and was prescribed a bioidentical compounded thyroid medication from Billy's pharmacy that helped me begin to feel better. With help from Billy's program, a wonderful

joint doctor, and an excellent pulmonologist, I have become able to function again.

"My multiple conditions have changed my life, and I will never be "normal" again. For me, normal is a very limited lifestyle to protect my body, but I am pain-free and feel infinitely better—a far cry from the better part of a decade where I thought I was going to die. I am thankful for healing and to Billy for putting me on the right track. During my entire ordeal, Billy was there for me, and he continues to help me today. He has dedicated his life to helping people achieve optimal health, and he saved my life. I would not be here to tell this story if not for him. Listen to Billy, learn how your body works, and protect it. I am living, breathing proof that you can survive with the right treatment and knowledge."

— Karen

The High-Fat, Low-Risk Diet

We learned earlier why cholesterol is a poor predictor of heart disease. Eating a diet high in quality fats is absolutely conducive to optimal health. Eating quality fats like animal fats, coconut oil, or avocado produces ketones in the body, signaling the need to break down fats and use them for fuel. This is how we create true fat-burning in the body.[1]

The body will begin to burn fat quickly, but it's important to **stick with it.** It will take the average person approximately 12 weeks to convert fully from burning sugar (state of illness) to burning fat (state of health) full time. My OptiYou RX Program teaches this process in great detail at our two-day OptiYou Wellness Summits, and participants are able to enjoy many of our meals, snacks, and desserts as a part of the experience. A high-fat diet in conjunction with intermittent fasting (a process where the first meal of the day is separated from the last meal of the previous day by at least 10-12 hours) is highly effective in creating that fuel source conversion process in the body. When it comes to food, always think: *fat first.*[2]

Science-Based Exercise

When it comes to exercise, it is important to remember that more doesn't always equal better. Studies from McMaster University in Hamilton, Ontario and other institutions show that even a few minutes of training at an intensity approaching your maximum capacity produces molecular changes within muscles comparable to several hours of running or cycling.[3]

It is possible that too much endurance exercise (such as distance running or cycling) can begin to burn muscle instead of fat in the body. These exercises use the same muscles at all times as well; there is no variance.[4]

Researchers from the University of New South Wales School of Medical Sciences determined that high-intensity exercise could burn three times more body fat than normal aerobic cardiovascular training. Participants' metabolisms remained elevated for 24-48 hours after completion of their exercise, creating a longer period of fat-burning in their bodies.[3]

Additionally, every exercise regimen should include some type of resistance training. This type of training, commonly referred to as weight training or strength training, uses the resistance from muscle contraction to build strength, anaerobic endurance, and the size of skeletal muscle tissue. That's right: weight training can help the body improve its bone strength.[5]

Success Is a Mental State

We always have to be mindful of our thoughts. Daily habits are key to creating permanent, optimal wellness and keeping our fat-burning machine in high gear. OptiYou RX is designed not only to reset your exercise and eating habits but also to establish new lifestyle patterns. Being successful starts with understanding the mind.

The first thing to do is eliminate negative thoughts. No more "I gain 10 pounds just looking at cake." Your brain can't take a joke from you, so you must take control of your thoughts and your body! Make your statements and thoughts count; be conscious of the image of yourself you create. The strongest thoughts you can have begin with "I am…"

"I am going to eat well today and do a solid 10-minute exercise routine tonight."

"I am going to beat this diagnosis by giving my body the fuel it needs."

Studies have proven that writing something down increases our chances of accomplishing it.[9] Journal. Write your goals. Then go achieve.

Sleep Is the Key

Do not underestimate the importance of sleep and recovery. Chronic sleep restriction **increases appetite** and **stress hormone levels,** affecting the body's ability to metabolize glucose. It also increases the production of the hormone **ghrelin,** which produces **cravings** for **carbohydrates** and **sugar.**[6]

Sleeping problems have also affected patients suffering from Alzheimer's, strokes, cancers, and head injuries.[10] Sleep disorders increase the risk of high blood pressure and heart disease due to starving the heart of oxygen many times per hour throughout the night.

Scientists have discovered that when a person is resting, the brain is consolidating recently learned data and memorizing important information. Dozens of studies have shown that memory is dependent on sleep.[7]

Rest affects fitness by allowing the body to replenish energy stores and repair damaged tissues. Rest is physically necessary so that muscles can repair, rebuild, and strengthen. During this time, the body recovers from the stresses of exercise, and the real effects of training take place. During quality sleep, natural growth hormone levels increase, which helps repair and build muscle after training.[8]

In short: get good sleep. It is essential for your health.

Change You Can Believe In

One of the OptiYou RX Program's biggest success stories was Todd. Despite being married to a traditionally trained medical doctor, Todd had no success in fixing the health problems that had plagued him for his entire adult life. Overweight, diabetic, having high triglycerides and cholesterol, sleeping with a CPAP machine, and on myriad medications for his conditions, Todd gave OptiYou RX a shot. In just 12 weeks following the program, Todd lost 53 pounds of fat and gained 17 pounds of lean muscle. He lost 10 inches on his waist and dropped from XXXL shirts to a size L. But Todd was happiest about discontinuing all of his medications and sleeping without his CPAP machine.

Since then, Todd has continued to live optimally according to the OptiYou RX Program. He keeps seeing continued results and has told me many times: "I'd **never** go back. I feel like I'm in my 20's again." Todd is the model OptiYou RX Program participant, but you can be, too. Success is waiting for those willing to take it.

Chapter 5 OptiNotes

- This book and a lot of the principles of the OptiYou RX Program go against what you've learned your whole life. That's okay, because it's backed by science.

- OptiYou RX is easy to understand and implement. It's a lifestyle program designed for a lifetime.

- Don't diet, don't eat less. Eat more of the foods your body needs, and it will tell you when it is full.

- Exercise, but make sure you're doing exercise that benefits your body. High-intensity and interval training mixed with some weight training and aerobic training are optimal.

- Keep your mind right. Be positive and confident. Journal and write your goals to achieve maximum success.

- Get proper sleep. It's important for every function in your body that you recover properly.

- If you are interested in obtaining optimal health, this book is a great first step. Your next step should be looking into the OptiYou RX Program. **It is a two-day experience that will change your life.**

References

1. https://www.ncbi.nlm.nih.gov/pubmed/28604374
2. https://www.ncbi.nlm.nih.gov/pmc/articles/PMC3945587/
3. http://dailynews.mcmaster.ca/article/no-time-to-get-fit-think-again/
4. https://www.ncbi.nlm.nih.gov/pubmed/20086477
5. https://www.ncbi.nlm.nih.gov/pubmed/20086477
6. http://www.medicalnewstoday.com/articles/307203.php
7. https://www.ncbi.nlm.nih.gov/pmc/articles/PMC3768102/
8. https://www.ncbi.nlm.nih.gov/pmc/articles/PMC3774423/
9. http://www.huffingtonpost.com/marymorrissey/the-power-of-writing-down_b_12002348.html
10. https://www.ncbi.nlm.nih.gov/books/NBK19961/

CHAPTER 6

The Five Pillars of Optimal Health

I mentioned in the previous chapter that the OptiYou RX Program is supported by the **Five Pillars of Optimal Health** that I developed. In this chapter, I'll talk more about these Pillars and how the OptiYou RX Program uses them to help protect your health, promote more energy, and get you looking and feeling your best.

The Five Pillars of Optimal Health

Pillar 1: God-Given Quality Foods:
You Really Are What You Eat

You've been given the wrong dietary advice your whole life. You've been told that eating low-fat is healthy, that vegetable oils are good for your heart, that carbs should comprise the majority of your diet. This is, quite simply, wrong advice that leaves you at risk for illness and poor quality of life.

So what *is* the healthiest diet? What will fill you with energy, help you burn fat, and leave you feeling energetic and fully alive? The OptiYou RX eating plan accomplishes all of this.

I've taken scientific studies and my personal experiences with clients to formulate the OptiYou RX eating plan. I don't call it a diet because diets don't work. Following this plan, you'll be eating great-tasting nutritious food until you are full. You won't go hungry because there are no starvation tactics. In fact, you may find yourself eating more than ever before, especially in the beginning.

The OptiYou RX Program shatters the myths associated with nutrition. It promotes a diet high in healthy fats as we discussed in the last chapter. It does away with the false warnings about butter and coconut oil, shedding light on the frightening truth about often-recommended vegetable oils.

Vegetable oils made from corn, cottonseed, safflower, soybeans, sunflower, and canola are loaded with omega-6 fatty acids, which cause inflammation. This is especially true when they are consumed in greater quantities than the anti-inflammatory omega-3 fatty acids.

Studies have linked omega-6/omega-3 imbalance to many diseases including heart disease.[52] Researchers presume that because vegetable oils reduce levels of low-density lipoprotein (LDL) cholesterol—the "bad" cholesterol—that this will lower the risk of heart disease. But we addressed the cholesterol myth in the first chapter of this book and explained that cholesterol by itself is not indicative of heart disease.

One of the real culprits behind heart disease is inflammation. Guess what high levels of omega-6 fatty acids cause? That's right: inflammation.

A study on Crohn's disease patients found that supplementing with omega-6 fatty acids increased inflammation, whereas omega-3 fatty acids reduced inflammation.[1]

Additionally, eating fish with a lower omega-6 to omega-3 ratio has reduced inflammation when compared to consuming fish with a higher omega-6 content.[2] Fish with lower omega-6 levels also led to lower total cholesterol, lower LDL cholesterol, lower triglycerides, and healthier blood flow.

Our ancestors ate an omega-6 to omega-3 ratio of 1:1. Most people in America today eat an omega-6 to omega-3 ratio of 15:1 or 16:1.[3] Here's some statistics about that:

- A ratio of 5:1 improved asthma, whereas consuming a ratio of 10:1 worsened the disease.[3]

- A ratio of 2.5:1 blocked the spread of malignant cells in people with colorectal cancer.[3] On the other hand, a ratio of 4:1 using the same amount of omega-3 polyunsaturated fats but increased omega-6s resulted in the uncontrolled spread of colorectal cancer.[3]

- An omega-6 to omega-3 ratio of 4:1 was associated with a 70% decline in total mortality from cardiovascular disease.[3]

- A ratio of 2:1 to 3:1 reduced inflammation in patients with rheumatoid arthritis.[3]

- Low omega-6 to omega-3 ratios were linked to a reduced risk for breast cancer.[3]

You get the picture: eating too many omega-6s and too few omega-3s results in inflammation and disease.

Disregarding their high omega-6 content, commercial canola oil and some other vegetable oils are also produced with industrial chemicals. Would you like a few toxic solvents with your dinner? I sure wouldn't.

You might realize that vegetable oils are high in omega-6 fats, but did you know that nuts are, too? Nuts (excluding peanuts, which are actually *legumes*) are healthy—in moderation. But eating too many of them can create an imbalance between inflammatory omega-6 and heart-healthy omega-3 fatty acids.

Hold The Mold

Coffee is a hot-button issue among preventative health circles. Should you drink it or avoid it? Most coffee sold in the U.S. is loaded with mold. Caffeine destroys adrenal glands, and chemical decaffeination is a nasty process that doesn't help much at all. Make sure your coffee is certified mold-free and goes through a Swiss-water decaffeination process—that means no chemicals are added and the process is carried out exclusively with water by using the principles of solubility and osmosis. To go from guilt-free coffee to actual health benefits, add some coconut oil and butter. Mix up in a vented blender for a delicious cup of coffee that's full of antioxidants and nutrients that don't even start the digestion process—meaning it's possible to enjoy even in certain types of intermittent fasting zones.

The Carbs You Need

Scientists have proven that humans can survive on purely fat and protein[53]—technically, you never need to eat a carbohydrate again to survive. But you should! Although we believe you should avoid what most Americans commonly think of as carbs—pastas, rices, grains, wheats, starches—vegetables are an incredible source of nutrients, especially *cruciferous vegetables*. Vegetables in this family include broccoli, cabbage, cauliflower, Brussels sprouts, asparagus, and kale.

Broccoli is very anti-cancer, and it can be inferred that other cruciferous vegetables share these properties. Broccoli can help prevent the body from switching faulty genes *on*,[53] so it is especially important for those with family disease histories.

You can learn much more about proper nutrition and quality foods in the OptiYou RX Program, including the best sweeteners that do not create a sugar/insulin response in the body, the one time you should eat fruit, and vegetables thought to be healthy that cause inflammation.

Maintaining Healthy Blood Sugar Levels

Pat was a diabetic taking 16 medications and 5 insulin shots to control his blood sugar and suffered from related issues such as blood pressure and cholesterol. Pat was overweight and fatigued. He had mobility issues, joint pains, and difficulty concentrating. Ironically, as Pat's number of medications increased over the years, so did his blood sugar and blood pressure numbers.

After just 2 weeks following the OptiYou RX Program, Pat's blood sugar numbers were so good his doctor told him to stop using his insulin shots. His energy was up, while his waist size, blood pressure, and weight were down. Pat said he felt like himself again and that he would **never** go back to his old habits now that he felt so great.

Pat's problem was following the standard of care in America like so many others. By his 12th week following the OptiYou RX Program, Pat had discontinued 14 of his 16 medications and his blood sugar numbers were 150 points lower than when he started—in the optimal range for the first time in **years.**

Pillar 2: Quality Nutritional Supplements: Price vs. Cost

Chapter 4 was all about why dietary supplements are not all created equal. You now know you have to watch out for harmful ingredients in multivitamins and make sure all your ingredients are absorbable. Just remember to go over the OptiNotes for that chapter when selecting supplements. My website is also a great resource: www.optiyourx.com. The OptiYou RX Program goes into great detail to differentiate between supplements that are quality/beneficial and those that don't contribute to better health. Remember: **the most expensive supplement is the one that doesn't work.**

> *"I recently had the good fortune of meeting Billy Wease. This pharmacist went out of the box for his clients in a big way! I've suffered with rheumatoid arthritis for years. After 26 years with a rheumatologist, I was becoming desperate. I saw 3 other rheumatologists but was only getting worse.*

"It was shocking for me to realize that they're only treating the symptoms, not the disease!

*"I've been on Billy's natural supplements for less than 1 month, and I'm so much better than I thought I ever could be! All of the rheumatologists said my hands could not be fixed. **They are amazingly better in just 4 days of taking the supplements.***

*"The proof was so dramatic. I now have hope, and I'm not looking at surgeries with no possibility of getting better any other way. **Please,** if you have this disease or any arthritis, it could be greatly helped with the products that Billy has created.*

"Billy did his homework. He is a pharmacist and believes in total body health. Does your pharmacist?"

— **Amanda**

Pillar 3: Water: Health via Hydration

Drinking the right kind of water is as important to health as eating the right foods or taking the right supplements. Unfortunately, even people who lead otherwise healthy lifestyles often neglect or are ignorant regarding this aspect of health.

Water comprises the majority of your body. The brain is 85% water, the blood 80%, and muscles are 70%. Water also has many important functions in the body. It acts as a lubricant for the joints, carries oxygen to cells, reduces constipation, helps regulate temperature, and much more.

Research shows that dehydration after exercise damages memory, attention, and the ability to perceive where objects are around you (visuospatial perception).[4-7]

Dehydration not only directly weakens cognitive performance, it also worsens mood, ruins concentration, and makes you feel like you're expending more effort when exercising compared to when you're well-hydrated.[8,9] Even mild dehydration in women performing moderate exercise caused these symptoms.[9]

Replacing diet sodas with water has been shown to aid in weight loss and enables the body to use insulin more effectively.[11] This means lower risk of developing metabolic syndrome and type 2 diabetes.

Not drinking enough water can also cause headaches.[12,13] In one study, 18 people who suffered from migraines (including two who also had tension headaches) received either a placebo medication or advice to drink 1.5 liters of water every day for 12 weeks.[14] Drinking the extra water reduced headache duration and severity.

But not just any water will cut it. Tap waters contain all sorts of toxins including chlorine, fluoride, and arsenic. Filtered water is a little better, but if you're seeking optimal health, you want to be drinking alkaline, antioxidizing water. (Again, for more information on selecting a quality water, visit www.optiyourx.com or use the OptiYou RX contact information on the site to talk to me or my team about your options.)

Your body is at its healthiest when in a slightly alkaline state. Early 1900s research by Nobel-prize winning scientist Dr. Otto Warburg indicates that cancer cells exist in a very low-oxygen, acidic environment. It can be concluded that low oxygen and highly acidic conditions contribute to cancer cell growth. What's the opposite of acidic? Alkaline—which is exactly why we want you drinking alkaline water.

Alkaline water is beneficial in many ways according to studies as well as Billy's clinical experience. When researchers compared the effect of alkaline water versus acidic water on bone health in young women, they found that drinking alkaline water resulted in less bone loss.[15]

Drinking alkaline water also reduces the risk of kidney stones and improves gallbladder function.[16,17]

Strenuous exercise thickens blood, straining the circulatory system.[18] Alkaline water reduces the viscosity of the blood post-exercise much more effectively than purified water.[18] Mice that drink alkaline water live longer than those that drink tap water.[19]

In cell culture studies, alkaline water acts as an antioxidant, blocking free radicals and preventing DNA damage.[20,21] In a study of rats with experimental diabetes, alkaline water caused a drop in blood sugar levels, triglycerides, and total cholesterol blood levels.[22]

Alkaline water is often freely distributed at health food stores and other businesses like my 3 Prescriptions Plus Pharmacies. Search the web to find a place near you or call 855-OPTI-YOU (855-678-4968) to learn about your alkaline water options.

> *"For decades I've had severe IBS. After meeting Billy and trying the water, I can say that I have now gone 2 weeks with absolutely no diarrhea, no stomach cramps, and my bowels have not felt this good in over 30 years. I believe the Lord sent me to you for this reason. I no longer drink carbonated drinks, and I drink close to a gallon of this water every day!"*

> — **Becky**

Pillar 4: Science-Based Exercise:
Power On the Fat-Burning Machine

Exercise is the best way to speed up results when following the OptiYou RX Program. When done properly, it speeds the weight loss process and helps rev up the metabolism to create greater energy and sustained fat-burning. Additionally, you increase your chances of living longer when compared to leading a sedentary lifestyle. It's important to understand that while 80% of fat loss is about healthy eating, exercise is essential for building muscle.

Exercise lengthens telomeres, the caps on the ends of chromosomes that grow shorter with age.[23] Longer telomeres are a predictor of longer life and healthier aging. In one study of overweight 68-year-olds, more time exercising and less time sitting was associated with longer telomere length.[23]

Researchers have found that light-to-moderate joggers live longer than most sedentary people.[24] A number of studies have found that exercise boosts mood; for example, a study of nursing home residents aged 60+ found that dance-based exercise can reduce the number of depressive symptoms.[25] The residents who did not participate in the program exhibited more signs of depression during the study. In another study of women with depression, exercise lowered levels of the enzyme Catechol-O-methyltransferase (COMT),[26] which is associated with depression.

One of the best-known benefits of exercise is improved heart health. One study found that 10 weeks of brisk treadmill walking improved heart and lung health in pulmonary hypertension patients.[27]

Another group of researchers demonstrated the importance of exercise in conjunction with healthier eating.[28] Ninety obese women were divided into 3 groups: one group who only ate healthier and did not exercise, another who ate healthier and participated in low-intensity exercise, and a third who ate healthier and participated in high-intensity aerobic exercise. Women in the third group increased strength and had the most dramatic drop in two heart disease risk factors (LDL "bad" cholesterol and fasting blood sugar).

A combination of stretching, strength training, and weight-bearing exercise such as walking strengthens bones and improves posture and walking ability while aging.[30]

Pillar 5: Rest + Recovery: Not Optional to Be Optimal

Many think of sleep as an inconvenience, a luxury they do not have time for. They're too busy working, taking care of the grandkids, or trying to get their small business off the ground. Maybe you're one of them.

Or maybe you just toss and turn all night, unable to sleep soundly. If that's the case, you're not alone. An estimated 50 to 70 million Americans have a chronic sleep and wakefulness disorder.[31]

If you visited my pharmacy on an average day, the number of prescription sleeping medications we dispense would scare you.

Lack of quality sleep increases the risk for diabetes, cancer, high blood pressure, obesity, heart disease, osteoporosis, and Alzheimer's.[32-35]

Inadequate sleep also increases the risk for car accidents.[36] A few consecutive nights of just 4 to 5 hours of sleep can cause the same symptoms as legal drunkenness.[37] A study conducted on nurses found that lack of sleep accounted for a 61% increase in needle sticks, 168% increased risk of crashing a car, and a 460% increased risk of being involved in a near-miss event on the road. If you ever have to visit the ER, it's best to ask for the freshest doctors and nurses.

Nighttime exposure to light (especially the blue light produced by our myriad electronic devices) causes melatonin levels to plummet. Melatonin is a hormone largely responsible for good sleep. The low levels of melatonin in people who don't sleep well are thought to be partially responsible for their increased disease risk. Melatonin is important for the immune system. It helps the body rid itself of cancer cells, explaining why people who are exposed to light at night have an increased risk of all cancers—especially breast and prostate cancers.[38-42]

Low levels of melatonin are also linked to high blood pressure.[43,44] Furthermore, melatonin deficiency is also associated with an increase in beta-amyloid plaque deposits in the brain.[45] These plaque deposits are associated with Alzheimer's disease. Additionally, low melatonin levels increase the risk for osteoporosis, heart attacks, and depression.[46-48]

Adequate melatonin levels can be intuited to promote healthier weight management due to the association between nighttime light exposure and increased obesity risk.[49] It also helps reduce inflammation in overweight people.[50] Melatonin increases levels of a healthy type of fat known as *brown fat*.[51] Brown fat is not associated with the development of obesity-related disease. Contrarily, its opposite—white fat—is associated with type 2 diabetes and cardiovascular diseases.

Six hours is the minimum number of hours of sleep we recommend, but more is better. Deep, restorative sleep can be aided in almost all cases by magnesium supplementation. My five-salt magnesium product is truly a miracle for some with sleep problems, restless legs, headaches, fatigue, and more. In some cases, quality supplemental melatonin is necessary. But we can help our bodies produce more melatonin naturally by having a set bedtime schedule, sleeping in a cool and completely dark room, and avoiding exposure to blue light, including cell phones and TV screens after sunset.

> *"I never felt like I got a good night's sleep before I started using Billy's magnesium. My restless legs and inability to relax kept me tossing and turning every night. The first night of using 3 magnesium capsules, I slept like a baby."*

— Joe

Let's Get Optimal

The OptiYou RX Program is a lifestyle revolution designed to help participants lose fat, have more energy, and conquer their health challenges. According to statistics from the Mayo Clinic, about 90% of diseases can be blamed on lifestyle choices rather than genetics.[54]

It's critical to understand that long-term use of drugs is not the way to obtain optimal health. **You** have the power to take your health back. Many of my clients have been told they'd be on prescription drugs forever or that their problems were inevitable simply because they were "getting older." In most instances, this is just **not true.**

God designed our bodies to be healthy. We get in our own way by not providing them with the nutrients, activity, and restoration that they need. The good news is: **it's never too late.**

Chuck joined the OptiYou RX Program at 84 years young. His results after 12 weeks following the program were nothing short of phenomenal. He shed 12% of his body fat and discontinued all seven of his blood sugar medications—some of which he had been taking for over **40 years!**

Chuck also gained 2.4% lean muscle mass, unheard of for an octogenarian. His blood pressure was markedly lower than it had ever been while he was taking drugs for it. He lost over three inches on his waist, and his joint pains disappeared.

Not bad for a guy whose doctor told him he was "just getting old."

*"Billy, you took something I thought was impossible for me to accomplish and helped me not only succeed—but put it in simple terms and made it **fun**."*

— **Chuck**

**To learn more about the OptiYou RX Program,
visit www.optiyourx.com.**

Chapter 6 OptiNotes

- The OptiYou RX Program 5 Pillars of Health are designed to help protect your health, give you energy, and reduce dependence on chemical drugs.

- Eat the right foods and the right fats. Review the Pillar 1 section regularly.

- Take the proper high-quality supplements to support and boost your health. Review the Pillar 2 section to determine where and how to identify quality supplements.

- Drink alkaline water. Review Pillar 3.

- Participate in high-intensity interval exercise with some weight training. Review the section on exercise in Chapter 5 and this chapter's section on Pillar 4.

- Make sure your body gets proper rest and recovery. It's more important than most think! Review the section on Pillar 5.

References

1. Nielsen AA, et al. Aliment Pharmacol Ther. 2005 Dec;22(11-12): 1121-8.

2. Sofi F, et al. Asia Pac J Clin Nutr. 2013;22(1):32-40.

3. Simopoulos AP. Biomed Pharmacother. 2002;56(8)365-79.

4. Gopinathan PM, et al. Arch Environ Health. 1988 Jan-Feb;43(1): 15-7.

5. Cian C, et al. Int J Psychophysiol. 2001 Nov;42(3):243-51.

6. Baker LB, et al. Med Sci Sports Exerc. 2007 Jun;39(6):976-83.

7. Shirreffs SM, et al. Br J Nutr. 2004 Jun;91(6):951-8.

8. Masento NA, et al. Br J Nutr. 2014 May 28;111(10):1841-52.

9. Armstrong LE, et al. J Nutr. 2012 Feb;142(2):382-8.

10. Corney RA, et al. Eur J Nutr. 2016 Mar;55(2):815-9.

11. Madjd A, et al. Am J Clin Nutr. 2015 Dec;102(6):1305-12.

12. Blau JN, et al. Headache. 2004 Jan;44(1):79-83.

13. Martins IP, Gouveia RG. Cephalalgia. 2007 Apr;27(4):372-4.

14. Spigt MG, et al. Eur J Neurol. 2005 Sep;12(9):715-8.

15. Wynn E, et al. Bone. 2009 Jan;44(1):120-4.

16. Marangella M, et al. Clin Sci (Lond). 1996 Sep;91(3):313-8.

17. Bellini M, et al. Minerva Med. 1995 Mar;86(3):75-80.

18. Weidman J, et al. J Int Soc Sports Nutr. 2016 Nov 28;13:45.

19. Magro M, et al. Evid Based Complement Alternat Med. 2016;2016:3084126.

20. Hanaoka K, et al. Biophys Chem. 2004 Jan 1;107(1):71-82.

21. Shirahata S, et al. Biochem Biophys Res Commun. 1997 May 8;234(1):269-74.

22. Jin D, et al. Biosci Biotechnol Biochem. 2006 Jan;70(1):31-7.

23. Sjögren P, et al. Br J Sports Med. 2014 Oct;48(19):1407-9.

24. Schnohr P, et al. J Am Coll Cardiol. 2015 Feb 10;65(5):411-9.

25. Vankova H, et al. J Am Med Dir Assoc. 2014 Aug;15(8):582-7.

26. Carneiro LS, et al. J Affect Disord. 2016 Mar 15;193:117-22.

27. Chan L, et al. Chest. 2013 Feb 1;143(2):333-43.

28. Okura T, et al. Obes Res. 2003 Sep;11(9):1131-9.

29. Lanza IR, et al. Diabetes. 2008 Nov;57(11):2933-42.

30. Park H, et al. J Bone Miner Metab. 2008;26(3):254-9.

31. Colten HR, Altevogt BM, editors. Sleep Disorders and Sleep Deprivation: An Unmet Public Health Problem. Institute of Medicine (US) Committee on Sleep Medicine and Research. Washington DC. National Academies Press. 2006. Available at https://www.ncbi.nlm.nih.gov/books/NBK19948/#a2000f7efrrr00018

32. Itani O, et al. Sleep Med. 2016 Aug 26. [Epub ahead of print.]

33. Wang K, et al. Endocrine. 2015 Jun;49(2):538-48.

34. Nesse RM, et al. Evol Med Public Health. 2017 Jan 16. [Epub ahead of print.]

35. Liguori C, et al. Neurobiol Aging. 2016 Apr;40:120-6.

36. Abe T, et al. J Sleep Res. 2010 Jun;19(2):310-6.

37. Shattuck NL, Matsangas P. Aerosp Med Hum Perform. 2015 May;86(5):481-5.

38. Nooshinfar E, et al. Breast Cancer. 2017 Jan;24(1):42-51.

39. Keshet-Sitton A, et al. Integr Cancer Ther. 2016 Jun;15(2):145-52.

40. Hansen J, Lassen CF. Ugeskr Laeger. 2014 Jan 20;176(2):146-9.

41. Dickerman BA, et al. Cancer Causes Control. 2016 Nov;27(11):1361-70.

42. Rao D, et al. Onco Targets Ther. 2015 Oct 5;8:2817-26.

43. Pandi-Perumal SR, et al. J Cardiovasc Pharmacol Ther. 2016 Jul 21. [Epub ahead of print.]

44. Sun H, et al. Curr Opin Lipidol. 2016 Aug;27(4):408-13.

45. Mukda S, et al. Neurosci Lett. 2016 May 16;621:39-46.

46. Zhang WL, et al. Oncotarget. 2016 Aug 9;7(32):52179-52194.

47. Amstrup AK, et al. J Pineal Res. 2015 Sep;59(2):221-9.

48. McMullan CJ, et al. Heart. 2016 Nov 2. [Epub ahead of print.]

49. Rybnikova NA, et al. Int J Obes (Lond). 2016 May;40(5):815-23.

50. Mesri Alamdari N, et al. Horm Metab Res. 2015 Jun;47(7):504-8.

51. Roman S, et al. Transl Res. 2015 Apr;165(4):464-79.

52. https://www.ncbi.nlm.nih.gov/pubmed/18408140

53. https://www.ncbi.nlm.nih.gov/pubmed/28596013

54. https://www.ncbi.nlm.nih.gov/pmc/articles/PMC2515569/

CHAPTER 7

Programmed for Success: The Secret to Shedding Pounds, Getting Rid of Stubborn Health Problems, and Eliminating Fatigue

We were each created with the potential for success in our lives, but each of us faces unique and serious obstacles from before we are born.

The fact is, we are **not** all created equal in terms of family health histories, stress in life, our available resources, and other factors.

There is nothing more important than your health. Without it, you cannot be a success. I could not agree more with this quote from the Dalai Lama, when asked what surprised him most about humanity:

> *"Man. Because he sacrifices his health in order to make money. Then he sacrifices money to recuperate his health. And then he is so anxious about the future that he does not enjoy the present; the result being that he does not live in the present or the future; he lives as if he is never going to die, then dies having never really lived."*

> **— The Dalai Lama**

Unleashing Your Potential

Chances are that you weren't born on a pristine farm with lots of fresh air, time to contemplate life and the creation around you, and the ability to walk amidst and commune with nature. Most of us are unable to eat directly from land that we tend and nurture, nourishing our bodies in order to help them flourish.

The human body is much more resilient than you may realize. It is constantly fixing itself. Your stomach lining replaces itself every 5 days. Your skeleton is always repairing and replacing itself. Your skin is detoxifying as you read this sentence. It takes energy and intention for your body to be its best for you. What have you done for your body lately?

I've taken what I learned from years of clinical success helping individuals to give you the edge for success in your quest for health and happiness. It's time for you to **take back ownership** of your health and wellness destiny. Following the guidelines in this book or participating in the OptiYou RX Program is doable, workable, and can fit any schedule. The more you invest in your health, the greater the potential dividends of energy, mental clarity, physical fitness, and hormonal and biochemical balance.

Out with the Old

Medical school trainers have a saying: "See one, do one." You don't need a medical degree to realize that humans are conditioned by the same concept. We eat, exercise, pray, play, and sleep as we have been trained to. To live optimally, we must **retrain** our minds and bodies.

It's time to discard many of the myths and partial truths about health and wellness you've picked up over the years. At this point in the book, you've already learned a lot. But learning and acquiring new tools isn't enough; you have to **unlearn** bad habits and discard the falsehoods that hold you hostage. For example, next time you hear a commercial about cholesterol-lowering products, you must be conscious of what you've learned: half of all people with heart disease have normal total cholesterol.

My goal is to impart easy-to-use, easy-to-adopt tools. As you've seen in the testimonials interspersed throughout this book, people **get results.** I love hearing those success stories, but the credit goes to the individuals who share them. I simply deliver the message; they are their own agents of change. I applaud each and every one of them, and encourage you to follow their model. The knowledge is in your hands; the onus is now on **you.**

"In 1977, at the age of 29, I was diagnosed with Crohn's disease and had my first bowel surgery. After surgery, I was prescribed Valium and Lomotil to attempt to control my bowels. I stayed on these drugs for about a year before quitting; they didn't help much.

"For several years, I suffered with irregular bowels, gurgling of the digestive system, heartburn, upset stomach, and intermittent abdominal pain. I was given prednisone to combat the inflammation, which caused me to gain weight, become bloated, and experience increased sweating. I was forced to eat a bland diet, which was hard to do.

"My symptoms continued to worsen. In 2005, I had a second surgery to remove more diseased bowel. The doctors put me back on prednisone, but I still suffered with irregular bowels and gurgling of the digestive system. I eventually decided to quit taking the prednisone due to the weight gain.

"About 2 years ago, Billy introduced me to alkaline water. I began taking a multivitamin, probiotics, and digestive enzymes that Billy formulated. My bowels became more regular, and I no longer experienced heartburn or upset stomach.

"Billy helped me, and I now own my own alkaline water machine and drink it exclusively. If I want coffee or tea, I make it with the water. My wife cooks all of our food in it. I can now eat just about anything without any problems. I have lost weight, gained energy, and feel so much better than I have in years."

— **Keith**

Change from the Inside Out

Who are you? A simple but intentionally provocative question. Genetically, you're a mix of your mom and dad. But remember, genetics just load the gun—your lifestyle determines whether the trigger is pulled. That's why the OptiYou RX Program is so effective.

Your health is not just made up of your genetic history. Diet, stress, spiritual life, mental perspective, and recovery time are all huge factors that play a role in what's known as **epigenetics.**

Genetics involves the DNA code that children inherit from their parents. **Epigenetics** studies show that harm or benefit comes from parental exposure to environmental factors passed down to future generations. In other words, if a mother is exposed to a harmful pesticide, it can have far-reaching consequences that harm her children and grandchildren. If a father's unhealthy diet makes him obese, this too can have epigenetic effects on his offspring and their children. On the other hand, healthy lifestyle choices can have epigenetic benefits.[1]

Think of epigenetics as a switch that turns genes on or off. The food you eat, the place you live, how well you sleep, how much you exercise, and the way you age all interact with your genes to activate or deactivate them over time. When a person develops a disease such as cancer, their genes abandon their normal state and are switched on when they should be off or off when they should be on.

Your environment and what you put into your body plays a huge role in your health. Just because you've been told that you're "genetically predisposed" to a disease doesn't mean you'll actually develop it.

How can this be? Epigenetics is **reversible.** Your lifestyle choices can govern which genes are activated or not. Certain supplements can also promote healthy epigenetic development such as probiotics,[2] folate, and other B vitamins.[3]

The First Step

Every journey begins with the first step. When you are adrift in the midst of life's hustle and bustle, finding a firm place on shore to plant your feet and take that first step can be difficult and overwhelming. But if you've made it this far, you've already got solid footing.

Chances are, you've been lost on a drive before. You probably checked Google Maps or asked a local for directions to your desired destination. It's only through this consultation that you can find the right direction and stop driving in circles. **The same principle applies to your health ventures.** I believe that by reading this book, you've begun to correct course and begin your trek to optimal health. Trust me when I tell you it will be liberating and fun.

But I Tried That Before!

You've already discovered why the dietary supplements you've used in the past may not have worked to solve your health problems. You need the correct, cGMP-certified supplements in their proper forms to get real results. Remember: **the most expensive supplement is one that doesn't work or harms you.** Poor quality gasoline will cause your vehicle to sputter and rumble. Your body is the same—treat it like an Aston Martin luxury car: fill it up with premium so it runs smoothly! After all, if we place that much value in a car that simply gets us from point A to point B, shouldn't we place **more** value on our one and only body? It's the vehicle that takes us through **all of life!**

I Already Eat My Veggies

Are you eating the right type of vegetables? Fresh produce, directly from the farm, not only tastes better, but it's full of enzymes and nutrients that are destroyed by conventional processing methods. How did your great-great-great grandparents eat? They ate organic before it was regulated or a buzzword. Their food was farm-raised and fresh. It certainly wasn't sitting on a shelf in a box for a year before they purchased it.

"Dead food is for dying people; live food is for living people."

— **Dr. Chris Meletis**

This is why it's so crucial to know what supplements you need to make up for the nutrients and enzymes you don't get through your food. The OptiYou RX Program can show you exactly what supplements you need—**and** which are a waste of money.

Your Success Story Is Waiting to Be Written

At the end of the day, nothing I have said matters without you. Because without your action, nothing will change. You can continue to feel fatigued and lethargic, to suffer from unnecessary health problems. You can remain overweight and have no luck shedding that stubborn fat. You can stay trapped in the vicious cycle of taking a drug to treat a health problem that depletes nutrients, creating another health problem to be treated by another drug.

Or you can take action.

Your success is wholly dependent on how far you are willing to take it. You can follow the advice of this book: schedule a consult with The 21st Century Pharmacist and a good doctor with an open mind. You can take your success really seriously, participate in the OptiYou RX Program, and take back your health.

Above all, my wish is for you to take back ownership of your own health and wellness destiny. Your future is yours alone to write.

Chapter 7 OptiNotes

- Without health, you can't be a success.
- Your body works constantly to keep you well, so fuel it properly and efficiently.
- Proper lifestyle change is doable, workable, and can fit any schedule. The OptiYou RX Program breaks this down to its simplest, easiest, most impactful components.
- Genetics only load the gun—your lifestyle determines whether the trigger gets pulled!
- Epigenetics are reversible.
- The first step is the hardest—and the most important. OptiYou RX can help you take that first step successfully (and many more after that!).
- Optimal health requires more than just doing the right things— you must do the **right things** the **right way.**

References

1. Li Y, et al. Epigenomics. 2016 Aug;8(8):1019-37.
2. Dasari S, et al. Clin Nutr. 2016 Nov 24. [Epub ahead of print]
3. Friso S, et al. Mol Aspects Med. 2016 Nov 19. [Epub ahead of print]

CHAPTER 8

A New Breed of Pharmacist

In today's world, it's important to make sure your pharmacist actually knows you and not just your name. It's critical that your pharmacist truly knows your medical concerns, drug allergies, and history of adverse drug reactions. Your pharmacist should be able to meet your specific needs and answer your health questions. A pharmacist is a highly trained health-care provider and should be able to offer you more than just your prescription and a quick review of the side effects.

When you enter a pharmacy to pick up a prescription, you're establishing a very important relationship relative to your health and wellbeing. Make the right decisions.

Selecting a 21st Century Pharmacist

When establishing your pharmacy home, look for these things:

1. Ensure that the pharmacy you choose has a regular rotation of pharmacists who will know who you are and be familiar with you as an individual patient—not just a name on a bottle or prescription pad.

2. Always fill any and all of your prescriptions at the same pharmacy so that they can work with your other healthcare providers to track potential drug-drug interactions and other concerns.

3. Find a pharmacist who is a perpetual learner. Your healthcare provider should keep up with the latest research and changes and advances in clinical thoughts.

4. Find a pharmacist who has done research and knows the proper supplements and their absorbable forms in the body—not one who is just peddling the highest-margin items.

Always let your pharmacist know what supplements and over-the-counter medications you're taking. If you can find a wellness-oriented pharmacist, you will have a tremendous resource for long-term health and optimal living.

When you select a pharmacy to dispense your prescriptions, you are literally **hiring** a pharmacist. Most people don't think about choosing their pharmacy that way. Usually, people simply pick a pharmacy due to some combination of other reasons:

- It's near their home or work.
- It has a drive-thru window.
- It's located in a grocery or convenience store they frequent.

Convenience is important, but quality of care is critical. Remember, you're really selecting the quality of the human being, their education, and their level of care—much like selecting a doctor.

Knowledgeable pharmacists are familiar with the side effects of drugs and communicate the risk to customers who've been prescribed these drugs. Unfortunately, these pharmacists are less common than you might think. Reacquaint yourself with some of these potentially fatal side effects by reviewing chapter 3.

A good pharmacist also keeps up with potential lawsuits against drugs. For example, they'll know about the lawsuit against the antibiotic Cipro (ciprofloxacin), which has been linked to a severe form of nerve damage known as peripheral neuropathy as well as tendon ruptures and aortic aneurysms.[1] Another example is the lawsuit against the type-2 diabetes drug Avandia, which has been linked to as many as 100,000 heart attacks.[2]

These are just the tip of the iceberg when it comes to lawsuits against drug companies for damages caused by medications. Over the last ten years, pharmaceutical companies have paid out billions to settle class action lawsuits and pay government fines related to damages caused by prescription drugs.

In 2010, AstraZeneca alone spent more than $656 million to defend itself against lawsuits involving Seroquel (quetiapine fumarate), a drug used to treat bipolar disorder and schizophrenia. The litigation stated that AstraZeneca did not disclose the drug's side effects of potential weight gain and increased risk of diabetes and encouraged doctors to prescribe the drug for uses not approved by the FDA. This was in addition to the $520 million the company paid to the U.S. government as a fine.[3] With billions of dollars tied up in drug-related lawsuits already (and many more on the way), you can see why it's important to choose a pharmacist who stays informed.

A good pharmacist knows when a drug can be used beneficially, as in compounding. Sometimes genetic testing can be effective in determining which medications will work best and cause the least side effects in a patient.

Focus on Learning

Becoming a pharmacist involves a lot of hard work. Most pharmacy programs require four years of schooling, meaning pharmacy students who earn a bachelor's degree before entering spend eight years earning their degree—although some students enter the program after just two or three years of prerequisites.

A pharmacist's education doesn't stop after graduation—nor should it. In order for healthcare providers to stay licensed, they must complete minimum hours of continuing education (CPE). The key word here is *minimum.* In order to renew their licenses, pharmacists must complete 30 hours of CPE every 2 years. A minimum 12 credit hours of accredited continuing education is required annually.

Don't allow yourself to be treated by professionals who only meet the minimum education requirements year after year.

A large part of what sets me apart in the pharmacy world is my pursuit of **progressive** continuing education. Pharmacists don't receive much continuing education (or formal education in their degree pro-grams) about dietary supplements, drug interactions with supplements, nutrition, or herbal medicine.

I'm trying to change things. I've been board certified by the Meta-bolic Medical Institute, a non-profit organization dedicated to educating physicians, scientists, and members of the public on biomedical sciences, innovative technologies, and anti-aging issues. I'm a member of an orga-nization known as the Professional Compounding Centers of America (PCCA), which allows me to keep up with the latest on compounding medications. I've also obtained a fellowship in metabolic and nutritional medicine and have worked to receive extensive training to formulate the most bioavailable forms of pharmaceutical grade supplements.

Individualized Medicine

My approach could be considered unique because I see each customer as an individual and not their symptoms. I'm willing to work with health-care providers to tailor each person's treatment to their specific, individ-ual needs. Compounding medications plays a big role in this approach.

Historically, pharmacists assembled many of the medications that were prescribed for their clients. Now most pharmacists count out a cer-tain number of pills from a larger bottle and ensure that they are properly labeled.

Compounding, by contrast, allows pharmacists to customize medi-cations for each patient. This can be advantageous when dealing with drugs that would normally cause side effects like nausea or are difficult to take because of poor taste or swallowing difficulty. Compounding phar-macies can make the medication taste better or create a flavored, liquid form. They can create creams or gels for skin application for patients who dislike swallowing pills. Compounding allows pharmacists an almost infinite number of delivery methods, from troches (small lozenges that dissolve in the mouth) to suppositories.

Sometimes medications are not manufactured in the required dos-ages, so a compounding pharmacy can create the prescribed dose.

Compounding pharmacies can also formulate drugs to be free of specific ingredients that may cause allergies in patients, such as lactose, preservatives, dyes, gluten, and sugars.

One of the most practical uses for compounding medicine involves pain management. Oral treatments for pain like opioid drugs are associated with addiction and side effects like constipation and nausea (which affects approximately 25% of patients). Opioids can also cause more severe problems involving the central nervous system, including sedation and cognitive problems such as poor concentration, persistent confusion, and delirium.[4]

Non-steroidal anti-inflammatory drugs (NSAIDs) such as aspirin, ibuprofen, and celecoxib (Celebrex) all come with their own list of side effects, especially when used for long periods of time. NSAID use can cause anything from common nausea to more severe problems in the GI tract such as bleeding, perforation, and intestinal toxicity. Chronic exposure to oral NSAIDs increases the risk of ulcers. An estimated 100,000 patients are hospitalized in the U.S. each year due to NSAID complications—and 5,000 of them die.[5] It's scary to think that some medical professionals advise patients to take NSAIDs daily without thoughts of natural ways to allow the body to correct the issue.

Compounding allows pharmacies to create transdermal pain medications absorbed through the skin to replace the oral drugs. These transdermal medications can provide customized doses and the ability to combine multiple drugs with different mechanisms. Compounded transdermal medications also decrease lower systemic absorption, reducing side effects and lowering the risk of abuse and addiction. The added convenience makes it easier for customers to use the medication properly.

One example of an effective transdermal pain compound is the pain-relieving topical gel made using the NSAID ketoprofen instead of oral Tylenol or ibuprofen tablets. Ketoprofen topical gel results in lower blood levels of the NSAID, reducing stomach issues and GI upset. Blood levels from topical ketoprofen use are approximately 60% lower than just a single dose of oral ketoprofen.

Bioidentical forms of hormones such as estrogen or progesterone can also be compounded. These compounds are chemically identical to the hormones produced in the body and are much safer than conventional hormone replacement therapies using conjugated equine estrogens and progestins.[6]

When a compounding pharmacist is allowed to combine estradiol (a form of estrogen) with natural progesterone, the problems caused by synthetic progestins (such as raising blood lipids or damaging arteries and blood vessels) do not occur. Bioidentical preparations of estrogen and progesterone also carry a lower risk of blood clots when compared with conventional preparations.[7]

Compounded hormones can be used to treat menopause, premenstrual syndrome (PMS), postpartum depression, infertility, and endometriosis. Bioidentical testosterone is often used for men who need supplemental levels of the hormone.

The beauty of compounding hormones is that it allows dosages to be adjusted for every unique body, a far cry from the conventional "one size fits all" approach.

Experienced pharmacists can work with healthcare providers to interpret hormone evaluations and determine the proper treatments and dosages for patients. Once they receive a doctor's prescription, the pharmacist can get to work preparing a bioidentical hormone formulation to exact specifications in strength, dosage, and form such as topical creams, gels, and foams, or capsules, suppositories, sublingual drops, and troches.

If you think compounding medicine can help you improve your health, find a doctor who is experienced in the field. If you don't live near a Prescriptions Plus Pharmacy, my staff and I can prepare and mail a compound to you with a doctor's prescription, or you can find a compounding pharmacist near you by using the "Find a Compounder" tool at the PCCA's website: http://www.pccarx.com/contact-us/find-a-compounder.

The 21st Century Pharmacist

I strive to be a modern-day pharmacist and go beyond the basics of the profession. I study the benefits of supplements. I keep track of which drugs cause adverse effects and the interactions and deficiencies they can cause in the body. I became educated on compounding and all its benefits. I know that improving diet and lifestyle can help you feel more energetic, healthier, and more alive.

My mission—the very reason I'm writing this book—is to help all people obtain optimal health and wellness through the best, most efficient means possible. I've devoted my life to studying ways to do so and sharing those ways with **you.**

That's why I'm asking you now: if you have learned something valuable about health and wellness by reading, please share this book with others. I need your help to reach as many people as possible so we can start a true **healthcare revolution.**

I want everyone to have the opportunity to lead a robust life full of energy, free from drugs, and without physical or mental limitations imposed by substandard care.

Everyone deserves the opportunity to pursue true, optimal health.

If you are interested in going deeper, learning more, and changing your health more radically than you ever thought possible, enroll in the OptiYou RX Program today or visit one of my pharmacies in the Carolinas.

You can learn more about participating in the OptiYou RX Program at www.optiyourx.com.

Chapter 8 OptiNotes

- Make sure you are a person and not just a number at your pharmacy. Your body deserves attentive, educated, genuine care—not simple convenience at the cost of health.

- Find a pharmacist who can discuss effective healthcare options with you, not just fill your prescription and tell you common side effects.

- Review the 4 most important criteria for choosing a pharmacist.

- Convenience has a **cost.** Quality provides value.

- Use Billy's example as the model for a 21st Century Pharmacist. Look for professionals with his qualifications and constant desire for more knowledge to better help you.

References

1. Eusebi LH, et al. J Gastroenterol Hepatol. 2017 Jan 16. doi: 10.1111/jgh.13737. [Epub ahead of print.]

2. Schmidt and Clark LLP Law Firm. https://www.schmidtandclark.com/cipro Accessed on March 1, 2017.

3. Drug Watch. https://www.drugwatch.com/avandia/lawsuit.php Accessed on March 1, 2017.

4. The Huffington Post. http://www.huffingtonpost.com/aj-agrawal/drug-class-action-lawsuit_b_10598018.html Accessed on March 1, 2017.

5. Branvold A, Carvalho M. J Gen Practice. November 27, 2014;2:188. doi:10.4172/2329-9126.1000188.

6. Mirkin S, et al. Maturitas. 2015 May;81(1):28-35.

7. Moskowitz D. Altern Med Rev. 2006 Sep;11(3):208-23.

About the Author

Billy Wease, RPh. • **CEO, OptiYou RX**

Billy Ray Wease, Jr. is a pharmacist with nearly 30 years of independent, clinical experience. Billy specializes in health and wellness. His mission is to change the lives of millions by helping them obtain optimal health, wellness, and fitness. He teaches people to eliminate the side effects and complications of prescription and over-the-counter drugs by choosing the right foods, supplements, and exercise to fuel the body.

Since graduating from the UNC-Chapel Hill Pharmacy School in 1990, Billy has opened three independent Prescriptions Plus Compounding Pharmacy locations in the Carolinas. In order to expand his knowledge and impact more people, Billy received specialized training from the Professional Compounding Centers of America (PCCA) and earned a Fellowship in Metabolic and Nutritional Medicine from the Metabolic and Medical Institute through the American Academy of Anti-Aging (A4M), which is supported by the George Washington University Medical Program. Billy always continues learning so he can keep improving the health and lives of others.

In 2015, Billy became the founder and CEO of OptiYou RX, a health education company based around a highly successful, life-changing wellness program designed to help participants transition to an optimally healthy lifestyle. The program's principles are rooted in Billy's *5 Pillars of Optimal Health: Quality Foods, Quality Supplements, Quality Hydration, Science-Based Exercise, and Quality Rest & Recovery.* The 12 class topics include the biggest health crises facing participants today, such as diabetes and insulin resistance, heart disease, hormone imbalances, gut disorders, and cancer. The program has helped hundreds across the United States, and it's only just begun.

Billy is currently working with several pharmacy schools to create an elective curriculum based on the OptiYou RX Program with an emphasis on drug-nutrient depletions, drug-drug interactions, and the insulin resistance epidemic.

To expand the reach and efficacy of OptiYou RX, Billy enlisted the help of highly-regarded doctors and researchers in the integrative medical industry to create four proprietary supplements: Multivitamin, Probiotic, Digestive Enzymes, and Magnesium. Billy believes these supplements create the foundation for optimal health based on many studies and years of clinical experience. These supplements are sourced from the purest quality ingredients and are manufactured according to the most stringent quality standards in the world, including quality control excellence, GMP operating procedures, independent certification of analysis, ingredient tracking, and product validation by the independent organization NSF International.

Billy believes that the health of millions of Americans can be impacted positively through education via the OptiYou RX Program.

Now that you know so much more about your body and the broken American healthcare system, you are in a unique position to take control of your life and become the CEO of your own health.

If you want to learn more about my Foundational Four supplements—what they do, why they work, and why I selected them, you can visit www.optiyourx.com/learn. There you'll find out more about each individual supplement, their ingredients, the process used to create them, and how they could help you take back your health and improve your quality of life.

To learn more about the OptiYou RX Program and how you can participate, visit www.optiyourx.com/me, email info@optiyourx.com, or call 855-OPTI-YOU.

I can't wait to see the amazing changes you make!

CPSIA information can be obtained
at www.ICGtesting.com
Printed in the USA
FSHW020429271018